T0031139

THE
MENOPAUSE
DIET PLAN

THE MENOPAUSE DIET PLAN

A Natural Guide to Managing
Hormones, Health, and Happiness

Hillary Wright, MEd, RDN, and
Elizabeth M. Ward, MS, RDN

RODALE · NEW YORK

The information contained in this book is for informational purposes only. It is not intended as a substitute for the advice and care of your physician, and you should use proper discretion, in consultation with your physician, in utilizing the information presented. The author and publisher expressly disclaim responsibility for any adverse effects that may result from the use or application of the information contained in the book.

Copyright © 2020 by Hillary Wright and Elizabeth M. Ward

All rights reserved.

Published in the United States by Rodale Books, an imprint of
Random House, a division of Penguin Random House LLC, New York.
rodalebooks.com

RODALE and the Plant colophon are registered trademarks of Penguin Random House LLC.

Library of Congress Cataloging-in-Publication Data
Names: Wright, Hillary, author. | Ward, Elizabeth M., author.
Title: The menopause diet plan : a natural guide to managing hormones, health, and happiness / Hillary Wright, MEd, RDN and Elizabeth Ward, MS, RDN.
Description: New York : Rodale Books, 2020. | Includes bibliographical references and index.
Identifiers: LCCN 2020006267 | ISBN 9780593135662 (paperback) | ISBN 9780593135679 (ebook)
Subjects: LCSH: Menopause—Diet therapy—Popular works. | Self-care, Health—Popular works. | Menopause—Alternative treatment—Popular works.
Classification: LCC RG186 .W748 2020 | DDC 618.1/750654—dc23
LC record available at https://lccn.loc.gov/2020006267

ISBN 978-0-593-13566-2
Ebook ISBN 978-0-593-13567-9

Printed in the United States of America

Book design by Meighan Cavanaugh
Illustrations by David Parmentier
Cover design by Mimi Bark
Cover image by Westend61/Getty Images

10 9 8 7 6 5 4 3 2

First Edition

To our mothers, our mothers-in-law, and all the women who have helped us understand that menopause is a new beginning

CONTENTS

INTRODUCTION

Every day, 6,000 women in the United States reach menopause, which amounts to more than 2 million a year.

No matter how startling, that statistic doesn't even begin to convey the whole story about the transition to menopause, which nearly always coincides with midlife. At any given moment, millions more women are also going through perimenopause.

Chances are you're one of these women, or you wouldn't be reading this book!

Menopause may be a natural process that happens to nearly every woman by the time she reaches 55, but that doesn't mean "the change" is welcomed by all women, or that the transition to menopause is easy.

Just to be clear, many women love the freedoms that menopause brings, including letting go of pregnancy worries, premenstrual syndrome (PMS), and painful periods. But far too often, women dread this life transition. Weight gain, hot flashes, and mood swings are among the reasons why women fear menopause, including the instantaneous, surgically induced kind.

Menopause is often associated with a loss of youth. That's reasonable, since the transition typically starts in your 40s. Though you may mourn your 20-something body (*we* certainly do!), wish you didn't have to spend all that time and money coloring your hair, and yearn for when you slept through the night without waking up because you're overheating, try not to dwell on what your life used to be like.

Here's the thing. It's quite possible that you will live up to half of your years *after* menopause, so why not try to be the best version of yourself right now and in the future? We speak from experience, of course. As two postmenopausal female health professionals, we know that it's possible to manage menopause with healthy lifestyle habits, as long as you're realistic. We want you to embrace what you can control, especially when it comes to body image. After all, the sum of your life is defined by far more than whether you still fit into your senior prom gown, skinny jeans, or that outfit you rocked five years ago!

Menopause and Perimenopause

We find that women are often surprised and confused about the transformation that perimenopause and menopause bring, and it's no wonder! Our culture doesn't talk frankly about menopause, and women often feel like they should suffer in silence.

Your first period launched your reproductive years, but there's typically no single event that signals the start of menopause, which is a long progression of changes from the peri- to postmenopausal years. In scouring the Internet for menopause details, you may come across confusing information that's not based on science. So, here are some facts.

Menopause is all about changing levels of hormones, which are messenger compounds that travel through the bloodstream and direct specific tissues to behave in certain ways. The hormone shift most associated with menopause is estrogen. Nearly every tissue in the body, including the heart, brain, bone, breast, and colon, has estrogen receptors, which is why physical and psychological changes occur when estrogen levels fluctuate, then drop.

The adrenal glands, located at the top of each kidney, make small amounts of estrogen, and fat tissue is capable of producing it, too. But most estrogen production takes place in the ovaries.

Ovaries hold eggs, which are contained in structures called follicles. The number of ovarian follicles declines during menopause and the ovaries become less responsive to two other hormones involved in reproduction, which are luteinizing hormone (LH) and follicle-stimulating hormone (FSH). LH and FSH regulate the levels of estrogen, progesterone, and testosterone in the blood.

Estrogen doesn't completely disappear after menopause. Though estradiol is the strongest type of estrogen, and is the primary sex hormone during the childbearing years, estrone is a weaker form of estrogen that's widespread throughout the body and remains present, even after menopause.

Aging is the number one reason for menopause, but there are other causes, such as having your ovaries removed, and premature ovarian failure (POF), which is when ovaries are prematurely underactive or inactive before age 40.

As ovaries release less estrogen, FSH and LH can no longer perform their usual functions. That's when you may start to experience perimenopause, which can last up to ten years. Perimenopause usually starts in your late 40s, which is when you may begin to have irregular periods. On average, most women are about 51 when they enter menopause. Technically, you are post-menopausal after you've missed your period for twelve months in a row without experiencing other causes, such as illness, medication, pregnancy, or breastfeeding.

It's important to remember that each woman is unique and will experience menopause differently. Some women have few, if any, issues, while others have more intense or longer-lasting concerns.

Your Diet and Lifestyle Habits Can Make a Difference

"You are what you eat" (and how much you move) is never truer than during the transition to menopause. Some of the most common issues during this new phase of life can be counteracted, at least in part, by your lifestyle choices. *The Menopause Diet Plan* tackles health concerns that result from the transition to menopause, including the following:

- Weight gain
- Hot flashes
- Sleep difficulties
- Mood swings
- Fatigue
- Changes in digestion
- Muscle loss
- Changes in memory and "brain fog"

- Osteoporosis
- Increased risk of heart disease, diabetes, and cancer

Sure, that's a lot of potential problems, but we've got you covered.

Enjoying a delicious, balanced eating plan, along with regular physical activity and other healthy lifestyle habits, eases the journey to menopause and supports better health. The last part of *The Menopause Diet Plan* is devoted to how to eat. There is no such thing as a one-size-fits-all way of eating before, during, and after menopause. What works for one woman may not for another. We get it. That's why we offer several approaches to weight control and a healthy diet in chapter 11.

We love to eat delicious and nutritious food (and some that's not so good for you, too!), and we've included dozens of tasty meal and snack recipes, as well as strategies for incorporating healthful food preparation into a busy life that may include working a part- or full-time job after staying at home for years with the kids, starting a new business, being a caretaker for a spouse or one or both parents, or any combination of these.

Join Us!

If you're looking for practical advice about eating and exercise that you can live with in the long run, you're in the right place. The good news is that you don't need to sacrifice the foods you love or work out like a maniac to feel better, sleep more restfully, and control your weight. And you can feel confident about our advice. As registered dietitian/nutritionists (RDN), we're trained to translate science into actionable terms.

Menopause is uncharted territory. You only go through it once, and it's difficult to know what to expect. That's why it's best to have friendly, experienced guides, like us, to help. Our approach is a blend of pragmatism, optimism, and humor, and is grounded in more than thirty years of experience each as RDNs, colleagues, and friends, as well as a lifetime of experience being female.

As moms who continue to juggle work and family, we're firm believers that perfection is the enemy of good enough. The goal is not to regain your 25-year-old body, but to be the best—and healthiest—version of yourself for the rest of your life. We've been around long enough to know that how you live the majority of the time influences your health the most, not what you do on holidays, while on vacation, or during the occasional dinner and cocktails with friends. We didn't give up going out and having fun after menopause, and we don't think you should, either!

Yes, menopause has a downside, but look at it this way: The rest of your life is waiting for you. It's time to take charge and live to the fullest.

Welcome!

THE
MENOPAUSE
DIET PLAN

1

WHY YOU NEED THE
MENOPAUSE DIET PLAN

> Before menopause I could eat anything I wanted
> without gaining weight, but after menopause I
> put on 15 pounds even though I hadn't changed
> my eating or exercise habits.
>
> —*Sue, age 59*

W hat should I eat for menopause?"
That's a question we've heard many times over the
years, mostly as part of a conversation that typically begins with weight concerns. Between the two of us, we have many
decades of experience helping people navigate weight issues, but to
be honest, prior to experiencing menopause ourselves, we couldn't
fully relate to the specific challenges this stage of life presents.

Though we understood that women's bodies change with declining estrogen levels and aging, we may have been somewhat
skeptical when listening to women describe how their usual eating and exercise routines were no longer working. Now that we're
both past menopause, however, these women's stories resonate
with us—and how! Just like the women who have gone before us,
we've gained some belly fat, fended off hot flashes, and dreamed
about getting a good night's sleep again. Our own adjustments to
menopause led to our search for the best diet and lifestyle habits

for midlife, and beyond. That's how we came up with the Menopause Diet Plan (MDP).

We're firm believers that it's possible to stay fit and healthy despite your changing hormones by prioritizing time for self-care, which includes enjoying nutritious food. While the MDP is about much more than what the scale reads, we're glad women ask about weight because it opens up the menopause conversation. When our mothers went through "the change," menopause was rarely a topic talked about much, even among women who were in the same boat. Thank goodness this is not your mother's menopause! We know a great deal more about women's health now, and the MDP takes full advantage of the scientific research on how nutrition and exercise influence physical health and emotional well-being.

Making Sense of Menopause Nutrition

There's a lot of information out there about what to eat. However, very little of it is unique to the menopause transition, which often starts in the mid-40s and lasts into the 60s. In addition, food choices aren't the whole story when it comes to menopause. There are several other issues to consider, and they are woven into the MDP, which is designed to prevent or manage health conditions that become more common during midlife, promote a better mood, limit hot flashes, and much more.

The foundation of the MDP includes five core principles:

Eat according to your body clock. Does this sound familiar? You skimp on food during the day and eat most of your calories at dinner and afterward, and you can't figure out why you're gaining weight and your energy is low. We are ruled by natural body rhythms that affect our health, and when you eat matters. Consistent food intake regulates your energy levels, heads off crabbiness, and helps prevent you from going overboard because you let yourself get too hungry.

Meal timing is one of the most important principles of the MDP. As you will see in the chapters ahead, managing meal timing is gaining ground for its role in weight control, regulating blood glucose levels, getting better sleep, and possibly lowering cancer risk.

Focus on plant foods. Plant-rich eating plans typically supply a balance of healthy fats, fiber, vitamins, minerals, and phytonutrients that help reduce blood pressure and LDL cholesterol ("bad cholesterol"), lower the risk of diabetes, and promote a healthy weight. Following a plant-based diet may be particularly beneficial for women before, during, and after menopause, in many ways.

Two of the most popular plant-based approaches to eating are the Mediterranean-style diet and the DASH (Dietary Approaches to Stop Hypertension) diet. Both plans regularly top international lists of the world's healthiest diets for their recommendations to eat more fruits and vegetables than the average American consumes, opt for whole grains most of the time, and include plant proteins like nuts, seeds, and legumes more often. Both styles of eating strongly encourage limiting added sugars and refined carbohydrates, but neither forbids them.

When followed closely, the DASH diet is widely regarded as an effective way to treat or prevent high blood pressure.[1] It's based on prescribed amounts of whole grains, fruits, vegetables, lean meat, fish, poultry, beans, nuts, and low-fat dairy foods, and it's particularly low in saturated fat and high in fiber. DASH is also rich in potassium, magnesium, and calcium to help with blood pressure control, and lower in sodium than the typical American diet. Lower sodium versions of DASH—1,500 milligrams daily—produce even greater reductions in blood pressure,[2] but may be difficult to follow in the long run.

The DASH diet is a lifelong approach to better health, and while it's not a weight-loss "diet," you might shed some extra pounds because of better food choices. For many people, the DASH diet is a big change to how they eat, because DASH suggests a specific number of servings of certain foods every day. See the Resources section in this book for more on the DASH eating plan.

The Mediterranean-style eating plan promotes seafood over poultry, and suggests less beef, pork, and lamb. It also allows low to moderate amounts of wine with meals. (However, if you don't drink, there's no need to start doing so in the name of better health.) Following a Mediterranean-style pattern reduces the chances for being overweight,[3] and women may experience fewer symptoms associated with menopause, thereby improving their quality of life. It also happens that this plant-based approach is good for your gut, lowers the risk of heart disease, diabetes, and cancer, and may help improve mood in menopausal women.[4]

In constructing the MDP, we blended recommendations from the Mediterranean and DASH diets that encourage ample amounts of whole fruits and vegetables, whole grains, nuts, and seeds to help you feel satisfied so that you don't reach for that extra serving or two of snack chips, candy, and cookies.

Our approach is likely higher in protein and lower in carbohydrates than the Mediterranean and DASH plans, and like these plans, the MDP encourages you to eat more plant proteins and seafood, as well as nuts, nut butters, seeds, avocados, olive oil, and other sources of fat that are healthy and satisfying. Collectively, our recommendations emphasize the most "anti-inflammatory" aspects of the Mediterranean, DASH, and other plant-based diets.

That's because most health issues that surface during the meno-pause transition and afterward, including cardiovascular disease, diabetes, cancer, and cognitive problems, involve inflammation. And, like all plant-based plans, the MDP promotes digestive health by helping to prevent constipation and nourishes the gut in a way that influences overall health.

What Is a Plant-Based Eating Plan?

Though evidence suggests that plant-based patterns benefit overall health the most, "plant-based" doesn't mean animal-free. However, you may need to eat smaller portions of animal foods while increasing your intake of fruit, vegetables, whole grains, nuts, seeds, and legumes.

So, what exactly does "plant-based" mean? At first pass, it may sound like vegetarianism, and it can be. But there are many forms of plant-based eating:

- A *vegan diet* includes only foods from plant sources, like fruits, vegetables, whole grains, soy, legumes, nuts, and seeds.
- *Lacto-ovo vegetarians* eat plant foods, eggs, and dairy products, such as milk, yogurt, and cheese, but no animal flesh or seafood.
- *Flexitarians* consider themselves vegetarians for the most part but also eat seafood, poultry, and perhaps, some red meat, or not!

(continued)

Despite the differences, all vegetarian-type eating plans focus on getting most of their nutrients from plants. Plant-based eating does not ban certain foods, as is the case with many overly restrictive fad diets, but rather encourages some foods over others. You don't need to be a vegetarian for better health, but you may need to significantly up your fruit, vegetable, and whole grains to achieve the goals outlined in the Menopause Diet Plan.

Curb carbohydrates and cue the protein. Research suggests that many menopausal women do not consume the protein they need. Based on scientific evidence, the MDP includes more protein than is typically suggested for women over 50. While it's important to include enough protein, timing matters, too. Eating protein regularly throughout the day helps to keep you feeling fuller for longer while nourishing your muscles and bones.

When you add protein to your eating plan, you may need to shed some carbohydrate and dietary fat for balance. We have nothing against foods rich in carbohydrates, such as whole grains, fruits, and vegetables. However, you may be eating more carbohydrates than your body can handle at midlife, and that can make weight control more difficult.

While there is no one-size-fits-all approach to weight management in the menopausal years, a recent large observational study from the Women's Health Initiative found that some eating patterns are better than others.[5]

Four dietary patterns were identified in over 88,000 women ages 49 to 81:

- Reduced carbohydrate (about 40% of calories from carbohydrates, higher in protein, moderate in fat)
- Relatively high in carbohydrate (about 60% of calories from carbohydrate) and low in fat
- Mediterranean diet (highest in calories)
- A plan consistent with the U.S. Department of Agriculture's (USDA) Dietary Guidelines for Americans (DGA), which is moderate in carbohydrates and low in fat

By the end of the study, nearly 20% of the women had gained at least 10% more than their starting weight. For example, a woman who started the study at 160 pounds would have increased to 176 pounds or more in eight years. However, there were differences in body weight based on eating pattern.

Women who closely followed the reduced-carbohydrate eating plan, which was moderate in fat and high in protein, were at decreased risk for postmenopausal weight gain. High adherence to the Mediterranean-style diet was not significantly related to risk of weight gain, either.

On the other hand, the higher-carbohydrate eating plan, which was low in fat, was associated with a marked increase in postmenopausal weight gain, regardless of whether a woman was at a normal weight, overweight, or obese weight at the start of the study.

Though there will always be women who manage to maintain a stable weight on any number of eating patterns, this study points to the advantages of eating a lower-carbohydrate diet during the transition to menopause.

No study is perfect, including this one. For example, the results were based on women with a BMI (body mass index, a measure of body fatness) under 35; none of the four dietary patterns protected women with a BMI above 35 from further weight gain. Also, most of the participants were non-Hispanic white women, so the findings may not be applicable to other ethnicities.

Control calories. Calories are often the "elephant in the room," largely because low-calorie diets typically can't last for long. For chronic dieters, the thought of counting calories can trigger disordered eating. We get it. The MDP uses calories as a guide for balanced eating plans. That's because calorie requirements dictate the suggested servings of whole grains, fruits, and vegetables to eat daily, as well as adequate protein, carbohydrates, and healthy fats.

While we provide some sample meal plans based on calorie levels, it's important to understand that estimating calories is an imperfect science. We offer ways to make an educated guess as to what your calorie needs may be, but all meal plans should be considered jumping-off points that may need to be modified as you follow them. Trial and error is an unavoidable part of the weight-control process.

Physical activity. No healthy lifestyle plan is complete without physical activity, which helps you burn calories, maintain muscle and bone health, lower diabetes and cancer risk, reduce stress, and so much more. We are firm believers in moving every day. Chapter 9 covers why physical activity and exercise are so important for midlife and menopausal women and how to fit movement into your lifestyle.

Let's Dig In!

No traditional eating plan, especially those designed for weight control, includes all the elements found in the MDP. The combination of a plant-based eating plan with more protein and less carbohydrate, meal timing, calorie control, and regular physical activity is stronger than the sum of its parts.

The MDP uses everyday foods, is a satisfying and enjoyable way to eat, and doesn't put a damper on fun. No food is off-limits, and it's not an all-or-nothing way of eating. You don't have to worry about having dinner and drinks with friends, going on vacation, or having to follow an unrealistically restrictive plan for the rest of your life. You fit the MDP into your lifestyle, not the other way around.

The MDP offers three paths to healthier eating based on your individual needs:

- Diet and lifestyle advice throughout the book that helps you adjust to the changes your body is going through during the menopausal years that can be used to tweak your healthful diet pattern. You'll find delicious and nutritious recipes and meal and snack ideas to add to what's already working for you.
- For those in need of a bit more guidance, a "balanced plate" approach offers an easy-to-understand template that translates the science of healthful eating for the menopausal years into nutritious food choices.
- For those who like more structure, a calorie-oriented approach helps you better understand what a certain amount of food looks like based on your estimated calorie needs for weight maintenance or weight loss.

The MDP plan is a result of decades of working with women, our personal experiences, and a deep dive into the scientific literature.

In the pages to come, you will begin to understand why and how the MDP is tailored to midlife women. Chapter 11 covers the details of MDP to help you easily put it into practice.

We're convinced that you will see the MDP as the way to fuel your body, have more energy, and feel better. Welcome to the "best" of your life!

2

WEIGHTY MATTERS

I want to be at a good weight for my health, but, to tell
you the truth, I want to look good, too.

—*Michelle, age 51*

Weight is often the number one concern for women before,
during, and after menopause. Aside from appearance,
weight management is probably the most important
issue during the transition to menopause because excess body fat
magnifies the risk for common conditions that increase with age,
such as type 2 diabetes, heart disease, and cancer, and it can aggravate hot flashes, a dreaded side effect of menopause.

Paying attention to your body weight may be a new experience
for you. However, given that government data suggest nearly 70%
of American women are overweight or obese,[1] weight management
is nothing new to most of us. In any case, discussions about weight
can be hazardous turf, fraught with landmines of emotion that
may be decades old and often infused with a perception of failure.

Let's admit that we live in a culture that objectifies thinness
and sets unrealistic standards for appearance, particularly for
women. If you look around, it's evident that women come in all
shapes and sizes, and it's the rare person who reflects the images
we see in fashion magazines and on social media. It's interesting

how we readily accept that we can't change our height because it's genetically determined, but somehow feel that if we're not as thin as we'd like to be it's completely our fault.

None of this is to say we should throw up our hands and accept that weight gain is an inevitable part of menopause, but it's important to have realistic expectations. This chapter will help you understand what is happening to your midlife menopausal body, how it affects your weight, and what to do to offset the changes without feeling overwhelmed.

Is Weight Gain Inevitable During Menopause?

Weight control will present a challenge for most of us as we navigate midlife. Research suggests, on average, that women gain about 1.5 pounds per year in their 40s and 50s, independent of their initial weight, race, or ethnicity.[2] In the United States, nearly two-thirds of women ages 40 to 60 are overweight, and almost half qualify as obese based on their body mass index (BMI). These statistics mean that women who were at a healthy weight prior to age 40 may start to gain weight and those who are already overweight may get heavier.

There are some women who ride out menopause and aging without putting on the pounds, but with the onset of perimenopause and menopause, even naturally thin women often start to feel the pinch of that newly emerging roll around the middle. Interestingly, while we were discussing this issue with an OB-GYN, she mentioned that it's these naturally thin women who often suffer the most distress about the appearance of belly fat because they've never had to deal with it before.

YOUR CHANGING METABOLISM

Midlife women's lives are complicated and often in transition on many fronts, and research to date has struggled to tease out the differences between weight gain related to age and that specifically attributed to shifting hormones. We do know that metabolism changes, especially once a woman is in her 40s, and it plays a major role in midlife weight gain.

Metabolism is the calories the body burns to sustain the internal work of keeping us alive (such as maintaining heart beat, breathing, and digestion) and represents 60 to 70% of your daily calorie use. These calorie demands for maintaining bodily functions stay fairly steady over time, but several other factors influence how many calories you burn, which may affect your weight.

As we age, we tend to become less muscular and more fatty. Because muscle tissue burns a lot more calories than fat, losing muscle leads to a slower metabolic rate, making it easier to gain fat.

Declining estrogen levels, which contribute to excess belly fat during perimenopause and menopause, compound the effects of muscle tissue loss because belly fat produces compounds that cause inflammation and contribute to the breakdown of muscle.[3]

Larger people burn more calories, even at rest, because they develop additional muscle to support their extra body fat. Men generally have more muscle and less fat than women, so they tend to burn more calories, which is often why they can eat more without gaining weight. Physical activity accounts for the balance of calories the body burns. This "external" work of the body can be exercise, having an active job, or caregiving, or a combination of these. Using muscles regularly also encourages them to "bulk up" to withstand force, further boosting your baseline calorie burn around the clock. Though physical activity can vary from day to day, it's an important way to burn more calories and may head off menopausal pounds. And you can forget about "metabolism boosting" dietary supplements. There's no evidence to support their effectiveness, and in some instances they are harmful when overused.

One study that aimed to clarify what's going on with weight and body composition during the menopausal transition is the Study of Women's Health Across the Nation (SWAN), a long-term study of over 3,000 ethnically diverse women. SWAN was designed to examine physical, biological, psychological, and social changes, including weight and body composition trends, during the menopausal transition. Investigators collected information on weight and body composition for eighteen years, starting approximately nine years prior to menopause through ten years after a woman's last menstrual period.[4] The results were as follows:

- Body composition analysis showed that about two years before the last period, the rate of fat gain doubled and lean tissue mass, mostly muscle, started to decline. This trend continued until two years after the final menstrual period and then leveled off.
- Body weight increased steadily from pre- to postmenopause, and also leveled off two years after the final period.
- As for ethnicity, black and white women had similar changes in body composition and weight; Japanese women lost some lean mass during the menopausal transition, but did not gain fat mass; and Chinese women gained lean mass and lost fat during postmenopause.

The researchers concluded that there's an increase in body fat through the peri- to postmenopausal years, and that body weight alone, generally reflected as BMI, does not present an accurate picture of what's going on inside a woman's body. For example, you may be at a healthy weight, but you may be losing muscle and gaining fat, which puts you at greater risk for diseases that become more common with age, such as type 2 diabetes and cardiovascular disease.

The SWAN data agree with a substantial body of evidence tying perimenopause with a more rapid rise in body fat and a redistribution of fat to the abdomen, resulting in a shift from a gynoid (the classic "pear" shape—thin waist, larger butt and thighs) to an android (the "apple" body—more belly fat) pattern of fat deposition. Research using radiology testing has also found more intra-abdominal fat—deep belly fat—in postmenopausal women compared to premenopausal women, which is unfortunately tied to an increased risk of type 2 diabetes and heart disease, among other conditions. Don't get us wrong. Body fat is important. Fat produces estrogen, which provides an alternate source of this important hormone as ovarian production begins to wane.[5] Body fat also pads increasingly vulnerable bones from breaking in a fall. We just don't want too much fat!

As we noted earlier, a loss of estrogen redirects some body fat to our middle and affects muscle tissue in a way that makes it more difficult to build and maintain. However, most research suggests that weight gain may be due more to aging than to loss of estrogen. Lean body mass decreases in both men and women owing to changes in hormones, as well as increasingly sedentary lifestyles.

Regardless of the cause, the loss of muscle mass makes for a slower metabolism that can easily lead to weight gain when we don't reduce calorie intake, increase physical activity, or both, to compensate for it.[6]

Body Mass Index: Are You Overweight?

The single best thing you can do to stay healthy and maintain a good quality of life in the menopausal years is to avoid gaining a lot of weight. But how do you know how much weight is too much?

Although not without its problems, the go-to evaluator of body weight is the body mass index, or BMI. BMI is calculated using your height and weight, and is considered a reliable indicator of body fatness. Though it doesn't measure body fat directly, research has shown that BMI correlates to direct measures of body fat, such as underwater weighing, considered the gold standard of body composition measurement.

BMI is important because it can help determine at what weight people over the age of 20 may begin to experience more health problems. It's figured using a complex formula, but anyone with Internet access can bypass the math by using an online BMI calculator, such as the one by the National Heart, Lung, and Blood Institute, found at https://www.nhlbi.nih.gov/health/educational/lose_wt/BMI/bmicalc.htm.

Once you know your BMI, evaluate your current weight based on the following definitions:

BMI	WEIGHT STATUS
Less than 18.5	Underweight
18.5–24.9	Normal
25–29.9	Overweight
30 and above	Obese

Don't like your BMI? Join the club! Before you start pulling your hair out, realize there are some limitations to BMI:

- BMI was designed to apply to large groups of people, not to individuals.
- BMI is calculated using weight that includes both lean (muscle and other tissue) and fat mass, so some people with a very high muscle mass may fall into the "overweight" range. Most people with a BMI above 30 have excess body fat.
- BMI is only one indicator of overall health; others include diet, activity level, and your personal and family health histories. We've all seen plenty of people who are thin but eat a poor diet and don't exercise, and many more who follow a nutritious eating plan and are active but are heavier than you would expect.

BMI measurement has its drawbacks, but it can also alert you to weight problems. If your weight is within the "normal" range, work to keep it there. If not, consider losing a few pounds. For instance, consider shedding 5 to 10% of your weight for better health. To find out how much that is, multiply your current weight by .05 and .10 to get a range. For example, if you weigh 200 pounds, a 5 to 10% weight loss would amount to 10 to 20 pounds.

You may think you need to lose more, but you should know that research from the highly respected Diabetes Prevention Program trials has shown that in people with prediabetes, a state that indicates higher risk of developing type 2 diabetes, losing as little as 7% of your weight may be enough to normalize blood sugars.[7] A healthier weight also reduces the risk for heart disease, osteoarthritis, and certain cancers.

Once you achieve a 5 to 10% weight loss, you can set another short-term target, if you want. Setting small goals and hitting them reinforces your confidence about long-term success and is much more important for better health than aiming for a larger number that you may never see, and don't necessarily need to reach. Just because you can't imagine getting your BMI below 25 does not mean weight loss of any amount isn't worth it.

Are Some Women More at Risk for Weight Gain than Others?

While the reality might be at least some weight gain for most women, others may be at greater risk for middle-age spread. The reasons why people gain weight over time are complicated. Factors that seem to raise the risk of obesity include the following:[8]

- *Age*: Risk of unhealthy weight gain increases with age regardless of menopausal status.
- *Race and ethnicity*: In both men and women, rates of obesity in American adults are highest in African Americans, followed by Hispanics, then whites. Asians may have lower rates of obesity, but also have a genetic tendency to accrue fat in their abdomen, which is known to be associated with a higher risk of diabetes.
- *Social factors*: These include low socioeconomic status, living in an unsafe environment, lacking availability or safe outdoor spaces for physical activity, high availability of processed food, and barriers to obtaining healthful food. Married or cohabitating people are also more likely to be overweight compared to those who never married or are divorced (maybe not surprising to anyone who's endured the potentially appetite-suppressing extreme stress of divorce, though the "divorce effect" appears to be transient).[9]
- *Low levels of physical activity*: Greater TV or computer screen

time has been linked to higher BMIs. Sedentary jobs and lack of a regular fitness plan also contribute.

- *Unhealthful eating behaviors*: Regularly opting for processed foods high in sugar and fat makes it easier to eat more calories than you burn.
- *Lack of sleep*: Many studies correlate inadequate sleep with higher body weight, possibly due to changes in metabolism or hormones that control hunger.
- *Stress*: Both acute and chronic stress affect the brain and trigger the production of hormones, like cortisol, that can affect your metabolism and increase urges to eat.
- *Genetics*: Obesity can run in families, although it can be tough to tell how much family influence is inherited or a result of learned habits. Genetics can "load the gun," potentially increasing risk, but lifestyle habits influence the genetic expression of those genes, thereby "pulling the trigger."

Additional risk factors for midlife weight gain include early menopause, lower intake of dietary fiber, higher intake of dietary fat and alcohol, and smoking.[10]

We'll address all these issues and more throughout the book, and we'll help you connect the dots showing how these life- and health-related factors collude to cause weight gain.

Consequences of Midlife Weight Gain

Midlife weight gain is a wake-up call. Without question, excess body fat raises your risk for a host of health problems, such as type 2 diabetes, metabolic syndrome, non-alcoholic fatty liver disease

(NAFLD), cardiovascular disease, stroke, cancer, and premature death. Higher body fat is a predictor of lower physical functioning, disability, and dependency (we'd like to take ourselves to the bathroom for as long as humanly possible, thank you!).[11] Obesity also promotes a pro-inflammatory state in the body, which is common to many chronic conditions.

What fuels much of this increase in disease that emerges with age are "metabolic disorders" that have far-reaching effects on overall health.[12] Increased levels of LDL ("bad") cholesterol and triglycerides, and insulin resistance that leads to prediabetes and diabetes, are common in the peri- and postmenopausal years and will be discussed in detail in later chapters. In addition, declining estrogen levels make blood vessels more vulnerable to the harmful influences of LDL cholesterol and triglycerides.

Many obesity-related diseases are also the leading causes of death in women, but equally distressing are their effects on quality of life. Modern medicine is increasingly able to add years to people's lives with medications, procedures, and therapies. This is great, but isn't it worth your energy to avoid these diseases as much as possible? Diabetes, which is largely preventable, can lead to blindness, kidney failure, and amputations. Being disabled by a weakened heart after a heart attack can make it tough to engage in your favorite activities. Obesity also contributes to reflux disease, urinary incontinence (as if a bit of urinary leakage left over from pregnancy isn't bad enough!), dementia, and skeletal and joint disorders, especially osteoarthritis, that can lead to more time spent sitting than enjoying life.

The Emotional Toll of Weight Control

It's clear that concerns about excess body weight and its health complications also take a toll on women's emotional health. We've seen it in action and we have experienced it ourselves.

Research has tied depression to obesity and higher calorie intake in midlife women. What's not so clear is whether peri- and post-menopausal weight gain contributes to increased rates of depression and anxiety, or whether the unique psychosocial challenges associated with midlife trigger anxiety and depression, thereby making weight gain easier. In many women, it's undoubtedly a bit of both.

At the same time that estrogen levels are decreasing, many of us are also dealing with age-related health problems, aging parents and their needs, "empty nest syndrome," financial fears surrounding retirement, or divorce. It's no wonder the menopausal years are considered a time of increased vulnerability for depression. One behavior associated with both depression and obesity that's familiar to many of us is stress eating.

Stress eating is the overconsumption of food in response to stressful situations or negative emotions. Stress can actually affect our appetite in both directions—decreasing appetite under acute stress (for example, a threat to safety, death of a loved one) and increasing our drive to eat under chronically stressful conditions, like work stress, financial pressure, or overwhelming caregiving responsibilities. Stress eating rarely involves carrots, celery, or apples. Stress eaters reach for delectable, calorie-rich foods that flip on the gratifying fat/salt/sugar switches in our brain. That often goes for wine, beer, and cocktails, too!

One review of the role of depression and stress eating in the menopausal transition highlighted intersecting influences that can collude to cause midlife weight gain:[13]

- Depression, menopause, and environmental stress are associated with lower estrogen levels.
- The combination of biological (lower estrogen), psychological (let us count the ways!), and social factors ("Why is this kid still living at home?") creates a hormonal imbalance that can induce coping responses like stress eating.
- Compared to premenopausal women, postmenopausal women are more likely to experience increases in appetite due to depression.

The researchers also found that depression was tied to a higher BMI in postmenopausal, but not premenopausal, women, and they theorize this difference may be related to the following:

- Premenopausal women may be more likely to experience a decrease, rather than an increase, in appetite when stressed.
- Because of lower estrogen levels, postmenopausal women may have more difficulty differentiating between hunger and other emotions.
- Postmenopausal women may have a heightened response to stress, increasing their risk for stress eating and weight gain.

In other words, lower levels of estrogen may exacerbate a woman's reaction to stress, raising the probability of turning to food for comfort. Stress eating appeared to be a strong driver of BMI in menopausal women, as high-stress eaters were more likely to be overweight and obese compared to low-stress eaters. On average, high-stress eaters had a BMI 5.5 points higher than low-stress eaters, which is enough to nudge a woman's BMI from a healthy range (18.5–24.9) to an overweight range (25–29.9), and from overweight to the obese range (greater than 30).

It's clear that midlife generates a serious call to learn non-food–related strategies to manage stress. You'll learn how to manage stress, anxiety, and depression in chapter 5.

While all the above focus on midlife challenges that can feed an expanding waistline, weight gain can also be fallout from having more fun or hitting your stride professionally. With midlife can come more disposable income, more freedom to have fun with friends (that often includes dinner and drinks!), and busier jobs that may require travel, which always adds a layer when trying to eat healthfully and stay active.

The good news is that, though we've become conditioned to "aim for a healthy BMI," losing as little as 5 to 10% of your weight regardless of where you start can improve obesity-related cardiovascular and metabolic problems (such as diabetes and metabolic syndrome) and reduce overall mortality.

What Does It Take at Midlife to Lose Weight and Prevent Weight Creep?

Before laying out strategies for midlife weight management, we want to present a few realities about calorie balance that may be hard to swallow but are worthy of discussion.

- Unless you're genetically blessed, once you get into your 40s (and maybe sooner), you can't eat the way you used to without gaining weight. For the most part, a loss of muscle mass combined with less physical activity is to blame. Muscle mass peaks around age 30 and then begins a slow decline that will drag your metabolism down with it unless you get serious about adding some strengthening activity to your life. The exception may be if you work on a farm, tilling your own fields, chopping wood, and dragging water up from the well every day, or if you have some other incredibly active job. And that's basically nobody.

- Eating patterns matter. When you under-eat earlier in the day because you're too busy or you're over-restricting food to lose weight, your good intentions will likely implode, resulting in overeating later in the day, and often into the night. Due to the influence of circadian rhythms on our metabolism (more on this later in the chapter), night is the worst time of day to play calorie catch-up.

- If you've made it this far being a "picky eater" who avoids a variety of healthy foods such as fruits, vegetables, and whole grains, it's time to try again. Taste preferences change over time. You need to fill up on something, and whole fruits and vegetables and whole grains take up space in your stomach without loading you down with a lot of calories.

- You probably need to sit less. Modern life makes it far too easy to kick back, but there's a significant energy expenditure price to pay for being more sedentary that must be acknowledged and reckoned with.

Much of what we've mentioned so far involves behavior change, which requires figuring out what's going to work for you in the long run. This is entirely different from following a set of restrictive diet and exercise rules that you'll eventually tire of.

Think Health, Not Pounds

Since the mid-1950s, the general approach to losing weight in the United States has been to dramatically change what you eat. There have been countless plans to choose from over the years. Some diets have recommended eliminating entire food groups (like grains, for example). Other diet plans promise to make it easier by selling you packaged foods so you don't have to deal with meal planning. Many require you to cut your calories way back, maybe as low as a 1,000 a day. Some diets are even lower in calories, usually as part of a medically supervised plan where you drink protein-packed milkshakes a few times a day.

Regardless of the approach, what most fad diets have in common is radical dietary change with the unspoken promise that if you just stick to the rules, you'll lose weight. This often generates the usual negative dieting self-talk: "If I just behave myself and stop acting so weak around food, I'll be able to lose weight." This kind of thinking puts responsibility for whether you do so or not squarely on your shoulders—if you lost weight, you were virtuous and good; if you didn't, you were weak and untrustworthy around food.

We've been nutritionists through three decades of weight-loss fads and have yet to see an over-restrictive plan stick in the long run. From an evolutionary standpoint, they're doomed to fail because they threaten the body's self-preservation instinct, and they don't focus enough on providing skills to support permanent change. Any dietary change that cuts calories will likely result, at least temporarily, in some weight loss. You likely know that you can't possibly sustain the weight you lose following a fad diet, or that you shouldn't lose weight that way because it's not healthy.

But somehow you hold out hope that the latest gimmick will be the one that doesn't result in weight regain. Countless times we've heard clients say, "Diet X worked for a while in the past" or "I've seen my coworkers lose weight on this plan." We understand the temptation of fad diets, but think about it: If at the end of following an over-restrictive plan you drift back to the lifestyle habits that got you into trouble in the first place, why wouldn't you gain the weight back?

Long-term change can be so challenging that it might feel easier to jump on the latest diet bandwagon. We implore you to start thinking differently. Stop dwelling on dieting and start framing the weight-control issue as one of developing healthier habits for the rest of your life. Behaviors that reduce your risk of developing type 2 diabetes, control your blood pressure, lower your risk of cancer, nurture a healthy brain, and help your feel physically and mentally better are the same behaviors that often result in weight loss. In other words, if you think about what to eat and how to exercise for your health, chances are that weight control might get a whole lot easier.

We're confident that our strategy may also help you avoid the psychological baggage that often comes with dieting. Also, focusing on the quality of life you want to have through this next phase—how you feel in your body every day, and what you want to be able to do—can be a strong motivator to make changes and stick with them. Take time to notice the positive physical and emotional feelings that come with eating healthier and exercising, including more energy, better sleep, less moodiness, and a calmer, more regular intestinal tract—things that have nothing to do with BMI, pounds, or calories.

What the Science Says About Lasting Weight Loss: National Weight Control Registry

Although many weight-loss programs can produce weight losses of 7 to 10% of body weight within six to twelve months, it can be difficult to keep weight off. Everyone's situation is unique, but a few factors are known to play a role in weight regain:

- Physiological changes that occur during weight loss, such as a decline in metabolic rate and changes in thyroid and hunger hormone activity, can make it tougher to feel satisfied by food.
- Behavioral changes can be tough to sustain. Boredom with food choices increases and motivation decreases once the novelty of looser clothing and better health wears off.
- Losing weight and keeping it off requires permanent, sustainable change, not "dieting," which is culturally how we've approached this problem.

In 1994, Dr. Rena Wing of Brown University and Dr. James Hill of the University of Colorado founded the National Weight Control Registry (NWCR) to help identify a large sample of people (currently over 10,000) who have lost weight and successfully kept it off long term.[14] The study is ongoing, and detailed questionnaires and annual follow-up surveys track the characteristics of weight maintainers and the strategies they use to sustain their losses.

NWCR recruits must be at least 18 years old and have maintained a weight loss of at least 30 pounds for at least one year.

Demographically, the NWCR participants have a lot in common: 95% are Caucasian, 80% are female, 82% are college educated, and 64% are married. The average woman is 45 years old and weighs 145 pounds, and the average man is 49 and weighs 190 pounds. Efforts are currently under way to diversify the gender, ethnic, and socioeconomic status of the group. The average BMI before starting to lose weight is 36.7—well into the obese range. Upon entry to the NWCR, the average member had lost 66 pounds (range of 30 to 300 pounds!) and kept if off for 5.5 years. About 45% of them lost weight on their own; 55% participated in group programs or in individual counseling with a therapist or dietitian. Seventy-seven percent can identify a triggering event that preceded their successful loss, such as a new diagnosis of diabetes or sleep apnea, joint pain, or an emotional event, such as being teased about their weight. Most had experienced numerous previous unsuccessful attempts at weight loss before finally being successful.

Common Strategies of NWCR Participants

The vast majority of NWCR participants used both diet and physical activity to lose weight; 98% report modifying their food intake, and 94% increased their physical activity. The three most common weight-loss techniques were limiting the intake of sweets and fatty items, decreasing portion sizes of all foods, and counting calories, which we discuss in detail in chapter 11.

For physical activity, the most commonly reported form of exercise by women is walking (great news, as all you need is a comfy pair of shoes and some time!). About 40% use the buddy system for accountability by exercising with a friend, and about 31% exercise as part of a group. Most impressive are the participants' reported quality-of-life scores after losing weight and maintaining the loss:

- Ninety-five percent of participants reported improvements in quality of life (both physical and psychological).
- Ninety-two percent experienced improved energy and mobility, making physical activity more possible.
- Ninety-one percent reported decreases in symptoms of depression.

This last point is particularly important. Studies show that regain after weight loss is significantly more common in people who feel more depressed or who are prone to uncontrolled eating, often in response to stress.

Habits of Successful Weight-Loss Maintainers

Despite some variation in approaches to weight loss, when it comes to maintenance of that loss, there are several common strategies among the "losers," summarized here:

1. The percentage of calories from carbohydrate and fat in the maintainers' diets shifted over the years.
2. Exercise remains a priority. Ninety percent exercise, on average, about an hour most days at a moderate pace, which is equal to 30 minutes of vigorous activity.
3. They limit television watching. About 62% of NWCR members report watching less than ten hours per week.
4. Members try to keep their healthful diet and lifestyle habits going through the weekend, allowing themselves a splurge a week, not a splurge all weekend.
5. Breakfast is viewed as important; at least 78% of members

report eating breakfast daily, which may help curb hunger and overeating later in the day.

6. Successful maintainers appear less prone to eating in response to emotional cues, underlining the importance of learning to manage our psychological relationship with food and adopting strategies to deal with emotions and stressful events in a non-food-related manner.[15]

7. They value sleep. Although many factors can affect sleep quality at this time of life (like night sweats!), registry members appear to have more "early to bed, early to rise" than "burning the midnight oil" sleep habits. They're also less likely to report short sleep, defined as fewer than six or seven hours nightly.[16]

8. Self-monitoring is common; almost 60% of NWCR members report using a diet, food, or calorie-counting app (doing so with pen and paper is just as valid), and 75% weigh themselves at least weekly. We discourage too-frequent weight checking, as it can lead to hyper-focusing on this one indicator to measure success. Registry members presumably monitor their weight regularly so they're able to address regain early in the process.

The criteria for NWCR participation requires having maintained a meaningful weight loss for at least a year, but how do they fare in the long term? In 2014, the NWCR published a follow-up study that checked on the progress of a subgroup of almost 3,000 participants. Most had still kept off much of their weight, maintaining 77% of their weight loss at five years (average 52 pounds), and 74% (51 pounds) at ten years. Most impressive is that over 88% had maintained at least a 10% loss, which is tied to significantly reduced rates of chronic diseases like diabetes. Not surprisingly, behaviors tied to weight regain were exercising less, eating more fatty foods, creeping portions sizes, and falling back into stress-related eating behaviors. Regainers were also less likely to monitor their weight. All this may sound very familiar to anyone who's lost and regained weight in the past.

It's clear that NWCR members spend a substantial amount of time and energy on managing their eating and activity, and they strive to be as consistent as possible. When they begin to regain weight, it is most likely to happen in the early stages of maintenance and is most often associated with drifting away from these strategies. On the positive side, members report that it gets easier to maintain weight loss over time. Once they've maintained a weight loss for two to five years, their chances of long-term success increase greatly.[17]

Take-Home Lessons from Successful Losers

Keeping weight off is certainly challenging, but not impossible. It often requires some support from another person (a partner, coach, counselor, or exercise buddy) or a group.

Research suggests that face-to-face support is best, but some may find what they need from an online weight-loss program or smartphone app, or support from a RDN or other health professional or counselor. Be wary of online chat rooms. They can be helpful, but they can also be breeding grounds for misinformation, particularly if they're not monitored by a licensed health professional.

Maintaining your weight loss may be even more challenging, as it requires swimming upstream against social norms that make it easy to eat out too often, fall victim to portion distortion, or spend too much time in front of the TV, computer, or phone. Preparing more of your own food and getting regular physical activity take time, which means priorities may need to shift.

EATING PATTERN MATTERS: UNDERSTANDING CIRCADIAN RHYTHMS

It's long been recognized that night-shift workers are prone to being overweight. In our experience, people who struggle with their weight often eat too little during the day and too much at night.

To better understand how meal timing may help or harm the process, obesity researchers have begun to analyze how eating patterns interact with our natural biological 24-hour shifts in hormones, metabolism, and cell and organ function, referred to as circadian rhythms. Nearly all living things have circadian rhythms, and these around-the-clock changes in cell function, physiology, and behavior drive sleep and activity patterns, and are influenced by exposure to light and darkness and by daily patterns of eating and fasting. These fascinating physiologic swings fine-tune the function of most of our organ systems, including our digestion, metabolism, immune system, reproduction, endocrine (hormone), and cardiovascular systems, as well as several regions of the brain.[18] Given all this involvement, it's easy to imagine that *when* we eat might affect how our metabolism responds to food.

Circadian rhythms have influenced eating and fasting patterns throughout all of human history. Simply put, our metabolism functions differently based on time of day: We are primed to metabolize and store nutrients optimally during the daylight, which we can draw on during the after-dark fasting hours, when the body is focused on rest and repair. With the advent of electricity, however, access to light after dark has increased our hours of eating and has robbed us of some of these important fasting hours, triggering circadian rhythm disruption.

We're now beginning to understand how eating at night can mess with metabolism and increase our risk of disease. Here's how it works. Blood glucose regulation is strongly influenced by our circadian rhythms. These rhythms regulate food intake, calorie burning, and hormones that affect how the body utilizes blood glucose, which comes primarily from eating carbohydrates. The main hormone involved here is insulin, which is secreted by the pancreas in response to the presence of glucose in the blood after eating. Insulin's job is to "unlock" our cells so glucose can exit the blood and enter the cells, providing them with a source of fuel.

Insulin also stimulates the release of other nutrient-storing "growth hormones" that tell nutrients from the foods we ate where to go and what to do. All these functions are anabolic, which literally means "to build body cells up." Insulin fuels cells with glucose and helps store what the cells don't need at the moment as reserves, including as body fat. This is great if you're a Stone Age woman trying to survive a famine, but it's not so beneficial for a modern menopausal woman with access to a plentiful food supply well into the evening. In a nutshell, insulin is all about storing fuel, and when insulin is circulating in the blood late into the night, it can inhibit our body's ability to burn stored fat as fuel the way it's supposed to during an overnight fast.

Now let's circle back to circadian rhythms. It appears the body is more sensitive to insulin when the sun is up, but more resistant to it at night. This means eating more food, particularly carbohydrates, earlier in the day may reduce the amount of insulin needed to regulate your blood glucose, lowering your body's exposure to insulin and other fat-storing hormones.[19] But the opposite is also true: Skipping out on adequate eating early in the day (or, like many women, being a good "dieter" until about 4 p.m.!) often leads to overeating at night when your hunger finally catches up with you. The result? Higher circulating levels of insulin and other fat-storing hormones at a time of the day when your circadian rhythms expect you to be fasting and burning off body fat. This also places additional strain on your pancreas by making it work harder to regulate glucose from larger meals.

Circadian rhythms appear to influence weight-loss success. One study divided 93 overweight and obese women into two different 1,400-calorie meal plans for 12 weeks. Both plans had the same carbohydrate, protein, and fat content. Half the women ate 700 calories at breakfast, 500 calories at lunch, and 200 calories at dinner. The other half ate 200 calories for breakfast, 500 calories at lunch, and 700 calories at dinner. All the women lost weight, but the big-breakfast group shed nearly three times as much weight—11% as compared to 4% for those who ate more at dinner.[20]

While there are clearly people who can eat at any time of day without consequence, it seems prudent to explore all strategies for easier weight control. It's worth noting that circadian cycles also wane with age, likely contributing to mid- and late-life weight gain. The bottom line is this: Regardless of any affect eating later may have on your metabolism, there's little downside to limiting the number of hours you spend each day cramming in calories.

MINDFUL EATING

We've covered strategies that help people lose weight and keep it off, and how eating patterns are an important part of the picture.

But *how* we approach healthful eating for weight management may be the most important factor—and the biggest nut to crack—as it strongly influences the food choices we make, and our ability to view eating as a natural process that can be planned for and managed, not something "bad" to be avoided.

Here are some of the most common misconceptions about food that women have, based on our experience:

- Foods are either "good" or "bad." Natural, lightly processed foods, like fresh fruits, vegetables, whole grains, poultry, seafood, nuts, seeds, and legumes, gleam with virtue while sweets, salty snacks, highly processed foods, and meats are often deemed bad for your health in any amount.
- Healthful eating is an "all-or-nothing" activity that must be done perfectly to be worth it.
- If you enjoy a food that isn't "good for you," that means you've "cheated."
- Eating a low-calorie breakfast and lunch is a good way to stay on track with your diet through the day—until the midafternoon hungry horrors set in, that is!
- If you just stick to "the plan," eventually you'll stop desiring your favorite foods.

Now let's reframe this thinking based on some realities about nutrition and our natural relationship with food:

- Individual foods don't affect any aspect of your health unless you have a food allergy.
- Food is not good or bad. It's what you eat most of the time that matters.
- Healthful eating does not require perfection. The goal is a

better, more consistent eating pattern that does your body good while including reasonable portions of foods for fun just because they taste good.

- Portion sizes determine the impact of any food on health and calorie balance. Incorporating foods you enjoy into your eating routine can help avoid feelings of deprivation and keep cravings at bay. Who hasn't learned the hard way that over-restricting often backfires?

- You are not defined by the foods you eat. We hate the idea of "cheating," which is way too judgmental for us. Humans are supposed to like food! It's all about choices. As long as your core eating habits are basically healthy, you can include small amounts of any food in your diet.

- If you eat 250 calories for breakfast, and 300 calories for lunch (we're looking at you, low-cal frozen meal), why wouldn't you be starving by 4 p.m.? Respecting your hunger by eating substantially earlier in the day can help guard against overeating at night.

- You will never stop enjoying tasty food. Access matters. Actively decide which foods are good options to have on hand and which ones you're better off enjoying outside your home.

- We all associate food (and drink!) with relaxation to some degree, but try to figure out if you're using food for stress management. If this sounds like you, it's important to learn non-food-related techniques to deal with stress, such as exercise, meditation, or talk therapy.

These thoughts just skim the surface of dealing with emotions around eating. There are many great books and online resources about mindful and intuitive eating. We've included one of our favorites in the Resources section. Learning to take much of the judgment around eating out of the equation is step one in shaking off dieting mentality and developing a healthy relationship with food during the peri- and postmenopausal years.

Coping with Lapses

Life events, as well as the holidays, vacations, and work travel, can veer you off course from healthy eating. These are off-schedule events when you may want to practice some mindfulness about eating but accept that what's most important is to regroup with your usual habits the next day or when you return home. But some lapses are common, so it's worth developing strategies to navigate them:

- Suppose you overate at a restaurant—maybe you were overly hungry when you got there. Next time, have a midafternoon snack with carbohydrate and protein, and eat a piece of fruit on the way to the restaurant to make it easier to order healthier options. (Also, be careful with whom you dine. Dining with overeaters may make it feel okay to step out of your healthy habits.)
- If you stopped for takeout on the way home from work, maybe it was because you skipped your usual Sunday trip to the supermarket. Schedule your food shopping on a weekly basis.
- If you grabbed a snack from the vending

(continued)

machine, remind yourself how important it is to bring a snack from home. Tuck one into your bag tonight before you go to bed!

- If you skipped breakfast because you were running late and, as a result, overindulged at lunch, set your clock a few minutes earlier so you have more time in the morning to fit it in.

- If you typically don't eat enough fruits and vegetables during the day, stock up on produce at the grocery store and pack it with your lunch and snacks. Store them where you can see them. Studies show that we're more likely to eat what's in front of us, so keep that apple or banana right on your desk at work and a fruit bowl on the kitchen counter.

- If you ended up eating cookies, chips, or ice cream in front of the TV after dinner, be realistic about having easy access to them in the house. These fun foods are out there in the world where you'll get your chance to enjoy them. Instead, try some fruit, a cup of herbal tea, or a piece of gum while you work on deconditioning yourself from eating in front of the TV.

A Word About Body Image

As women age, their bodies change. No matter how much we've prioritized healthy living by eating right and exercising, life leaves its imprint. Be it stretch marks from pregnancy (we've had three kids each, so we know!), wrinkles from not using enough sunscreen, or a thickening waist that seems unfair given our efforts to prevent it, approaching the perimenopausal years with the aim of stopping time is unrealistic. Yes, the pressure to look fabulous to the end is intense, but hyper-focusing on body image can chew up a lot of time better spent having fun and exploring new pursuits. We know, it's not easy. We find it highly therapeutic to complain about it to each other, and then to get on with the business of donating the clothes that will never fit comfortably again!

Accepting your changing body is also important for your emotional health, as research suggests that midlife women with a poor body image may be more likely to suffer clinically significant depression.[21] The goal of this book is to help women become the best versions of themselves at this stage of life, ready to enjoy or navigate whatever life sends their way regardless of how much they weigh or what size they wear. We continue to work on accepting what can't be changed; in the meantime, we are grateful for clothes with some stretch, treat ourselves to special ointments and quality cosmetics, and are comforted by the fact that all the women we know of the same age feel the same way.

Final Thought: View Weight Management as a Behavior Change Process, Not a Diet

The whole concept of dieting tends to psychologically bring out the worst in us. Women tend to be very hard on themselves. Have you ever had these thoughts when contemplating weight loss—yet again?

"I can't do this. I've tried this so many times before and failed. Why bother?"

"My body is just incapable of weight loss. I'm addicted to food and no diet is going to fix that."

"I have no self-control. I always seem to drift back to this place that gets me into trouble."

"I'm so uncoordinated. Exercise is so uncomfortable for me."

This is just a sampling of some of the negative self-talk we've heard over the years (usually prefaced with "I know this is bad but . . .") by women who are unhappy with their weight. It's easy to see how you could focus on past failures, but the good news is that previous weight-loss attempts can be valuable sources of information; most often they tell us what doesn't work long term, but also what was helpful. These historical weight-loss lessons can go into your tool kit of skills and strategies that may help you achieve and maintain the healthiest weight possible without forgoing a healthy relationship with tasty food.

Trying so hard at something, only to be unsuccessful in the long run, hurts! But you have two choices: (1) Keep doing what you're doing and become increasingly unhappy about the state of your health or quality of life, or (2) start chipping away at it in a positive direction. That's what the Menopause Diet Plan guides you to do.

Throughout this book we'll be encouraging you to embrace the "80/20" approach to healthful eating. We aren't perfect eaters, and you shouldn't aim to be either. We care about what we do most of the time, not some of the time. All foods truly can fit.

As for how to eat to support weight control, we pull it all together for you in delicious and nutritious eating plans at the end of the book. Chapter 11 fleshes out several options for implementing the Menopause Diet Plan based on your personal goals.

3

TAKE YOUR HEALTH TO HEART

My cholesterol was great until I got past menopause. I didn't want to go on medication, so I changed my diet and tried to increase my walking, which seems to be helping.

—Kathy, age 57

t's easy to believe that heart health is more of a man's issue than it is a woman's. And that's true, up to a point. Heart problems are generally less common in women until the menopause transition, which intensifies the likelihood for issues with your heart and blood vessels.[1]

In fact, more women in the United States die from heart disease than from any other cause.[2] The silver lining is that problems with the heart and brain typically take years to develop, are often preventable, and are manageable. There are many ways to keep your heart healthy before, during, and after menopause, and the sooner you start, the better.

Heart Health Terms, Defined

Cardiovascular disease is an umbrella term that includes coronary heart disease (CHD), heart attack, and stroke, as well as heart failure, arrhythmia (abnormal heart rhythm), and heart valve problems.

Coronary heart disease, also called heart disease, refers to blocked arteries that may result in a heart attack or stroke. Atherosclerosis is the actual build-up of fatty plaques in arteries that can limit or obstruct blood flow. These arterial "road blocks" most often originate in the coronary arteries, which are large vessels located closest to the heart.

Plaque is problematic because it thickens and stiffens arteries so they can't relax and expand as readily to promote proper blood flow. Plaque can also rupture and trigger a blood clot, which may further narrow a blood vessel or completely impede it. When blood is blocked from getting to the heart, a heart attack occurs. When blood can't get to the brain, that's a stroke. (Read more about brain health in chapter 5.)

The accumulation of plaque in arteries farther away from the heart is called peripheral vascular disease (PVD). PVD typically affects the legs and feet, but it can also limit blood flow to the arms. People with heart disease may also have PVD.[3]

Heart problems affect men and women differently. While men are most often diagnosed earlier in life with heart disease, heart disease may hit women harder, and in different ways. According to the National Heart, Lung, and Blood Institute (NHLBI), women may be at greater risk for serious complications of CHD and for a condition called coronary microvascular disease.[4] Coronary microvascular disease affects the smallest arteries of the heart, preventing normal blood flow, and it can occur alone or with CHD or other heart problems.[5]

Menopause and Heart Health

Though menopause does not *cause* cardiovascular conditions, it raises the risk for developing them. Before menopause, women have less chance for developing artery blockages than men. At around age 55, the likelihood of heart disease increases at the same rate in both sexes. Higher estrogen levels prior to menopause may explain the difference in risk.

While it's not completely clear how estrogen plays into delaying the development of heart troubles, it may promote greater blood vessel flexibility and discourage plaque formation and inflammation in your arteries. In addition, reaching menopause by age 45 is linked to a higher risk of CHD.[6, 7]

It's likely that changes to heart health begin long before your last period. During perimenopause, decreased and fluctuating hormone levels are tied to having more heart palpitations, known as arrhythmia. Your heart may flutter, race, pound, or beat irregularly during a palpitation, which can last from a few seconds to a few minutes. In general, heart palpitations are harmless, but if you have them often, consult your doctor or nurse practitioner.[8]

Risk Factors for Heart Disease

Heart disease is probably not on your radar, but it should be, especially because of menopause. According to the NHLBI, 80% of women ages 40 to 60 have one or more risk factors for heart disease. Having more than one risk factor further boosts the chances for developing heart disease.[9]

The statistics can be scary, but if you've followed a relatively healthy lifestyle for many years, and you keep it up before, during, and after menopause, it reduces your chances for cardiovascular problems. That's not to say that all the bodily changes that come with menopause are completely under your control, however.

Discuss your heart health with your doctor or nurse practitioner, who should fully evaluate your chances for heart disease. It's never too late, or too early, to take better care of your heart.

Inflammation and Heart Disease

Inflammation is a hot topic, especially as it relates to heart health. You may know inflammation as the rapid response of your immune system to an illness or injury, like the redness surrounding a cut or the swelling after twisting your ankle. Such acute, or short-term, inflammation comes and goes and isn't regarded as a threat to heart health. Chronic inflammation—the type that persists for months or years—is another matter. This long-lasting inflammation irritates blood vessels, possibly promoting the growth of plaque, and plays a part in loosening plaque and triggering blood clots that cause heart attack and stroke. Smoking, high blood pressure, and elevated levels of LDL cholesterol contribute to chronic inflammation, while a diet rich in plant foods helps to fight it.

Body weight and belly fat. Perimenopause and menopause often result in weight gain for the many reasons explained in chapter 2. How you carry your weight matters to heart health.

Research shows that gaining weight in the abdomen signals an increase in visceral fat in the body, which is fat surrounding your internal organs. An excess of visceral fat is linked to type 2 diabetes, elevated blood pressure, and high blood cholesterol, which are risk factors for heart disease. Women who carry more weight around the middle have a greater chance for heart attack than women who are just heavier overall.[10]

Prediabetes and diabetes. Diabetes is a major risk factor for cardiovascular disease, and strategies to prevent diabetes, and its precursor prediabetes, are covered in detail in chapter 4. Consistently elevated glucose levels harm blood vessels and the nerves that control your heart and blood vessels. The longer you have diabetes, the higher the risk for heart disease.[11] Prediabetes, which is when blood glucose concentrations are higher than normal but not yet at the level of diabetes, is also associated with an increased risk of heart attack or stroke.[12] Fortunately, the strategies to control diabetes are also good for your heart.

High blood pressure. Your heart beats for the sole purpose of pushing blood through blood vessels from the largest to the smallest. The goal is to deliver oxygen and nutrients found in the blood to every tissue and organ in the body. As the heart beats, it creates pressure so that blood can get to where it needs to go. Blood pressure is the force of blood pushing against arteries.

Blood pressure results are given as two numbers, a systolic pressure over a diastolic pressure—for example, 118/78. Systolic pressure is the top number. It's caused by your heart contracting and pushing out blood. Diastolic pressure, the bottom number, is the force when your heart relaxes and fills with blood.

High blood pressure, also called hypertension, is when blood pressure is consistently elevated, and in the postmenopausal years it plays a significant role in the development of CHD, chronic heart failure, and stroke in older women.[13]

The constant, extra force created by high blood pressure creates tiny tears in vessel walls that encourage plaque to accumulate and to narrow the arteries. The narrower the arteries, the harder the heart must work to get blood where it should go, making the heart and vessels less efficient over time. Aging results in stiffer arteries, and lower estrogen levels may compound the problem of higher blood pressure readings in women after menopause. Weight gain may also elevate blood pressure. Excess body weight strains the heart as it struggles to move blood around a bigger body.

High blood pressure is often referred to as a silent health threat because it can take a toll on health without any signs. Get your blood pressure checked at least once a year, even if you feel fine. Normal blood pressure for adults is 120/80. If your blood pressure is above 130/80, discuss how best to lower it with your doctor or nurse practitioner, and with a registered dietitian/nutritionist (RDN). Depending on your health history, you may require medication along with a balanced diet and regular exercise to reduce your blood pressure and keep it within a healthy range.[14]

High cholesterol and triglycerides. Cholesterol is a fatty, wax-like substance the body uses to form cell membranes and to produce vitamin D and hormones. The body makes cholesterol in the liver and releases it into the bloodstream. Animal foods are another source of cholesterol for the body.

Cholesterol is part lipid (fat) and part protein, which is why it's called a lipoprotein. Two main types of lipoproteins ferry cholesterol throughout the body, and they differ in form and function:

- *Low-density lipoproteins (LDL)* are considered "bad" cholesterol. LDL contain a high concentration of cholesterol, and excess LDL contribute to fatty build-up in arteries.

- *High-density lipoproteins (HDL)* are known as "good" cholesterol. Higher HDL help protect against heart attack and
  stroke. HDL are desirable because of their relatively low
  quantity of cholesterol, and because they can remove cholesterol from cells involved in plaque build-up.

Generally speaking, LDL levels rise and HDL levels fall after
menopause, creating an unfavorable situation for the heart and
blood vessels. Type 2 diabetes, smoking, being overweight, and
physical inactivity also contribute to high LDL and low HDL levels.

The American Heart Association recommends all adults age 20
or older have their blood cholesterol, as well as other risk factors for
heart disease, checked every four to six years. When your blood is
tested for cholesterol levels, you should receive readings for total
cholesterol, LDL, HDL, and triglycerides.[15]

Total cholesterol is not a type of cholesterol. It's calculated by
adding levels for LDL, HDL, and 20% of blood triglyceride levels.
In women over age 20, it's most desirable for total cholesterol to be
under 200 milligrams per deciliter (mg/dl). LDL should be less
than 130 mg/dl, and HDL should be 50 mg/dl or higher.[16]

What Works for Us

My total cholesterol went up about 30 points about two
years before I officially hit menopause, then a year after
menopause it dropped back down 30 points. My HDL
stayed the same—the difference was all LDL. I don't recall changing things much, though, so I assume it was
related to hormones.

—Hillary

Triglyceride is another name for fat. When you eat a meal or snack, some of the calories from food that your body doesn't need immediately for energy are stored as triglycerides. The body mobilizes triglycerides to use as fuel between meals. However, excess triglycerides in the blood on a constant basis can contribute to the hardening and thickening of arteries. Very high triglyceride levels can also inflame the pancreas.

Being overweight, having a sedentary lifestyle, smoking, and eating a diet that's consistently rich in refined carbohydrates, including added sugars, and alcohol all increase blood triglycerides. Certain conditions, such as thyroid disease, diabetes, and liver and kidney disease, also increase triglyceride concentrations. Excessive triglyceride levels in the blood may also be a result of genetics.[17, 18]

Your cholesterol scores should include a measurement for triglycerides. A healthy level of triglycerides in the blood is less than 150 mg/dl. It's important to measure triglycerides in a fasting state because they are influenced by a recent meal or snack.

Smoking. Any amount of smoking contributes to clogged arteries, decreases their flexibility, and reduces HDL levels. Smoking may speed up the onset of menopause, which diminishes heart health by reducing estrogen levels in the body earlier in life.[19] It's not easy to give up cigarettes, but it's worth trying to do so for your own health and for the well-being of those around you.

Lowering Your Risk of Heart Disease

There are more than a few ways to lower your risk of heart disease, including the following.

Physical activity. Regular exercise helps protect the heart in several ways. Even just a little exercise can make a difference to your health, especially if you're inactive! According to the 2018 Physical Activity Guidelines for Americans, the many long-term benefits of exercise include helping to reduce high blood pressure, type 2 diabetes, and elevated blood cholesterol levels.[20] Physical activity can also counteract the effects of stress, ease the symptoms of anxiety, and perhaps reduce the risk for depression and anxiety, which may contribute to cardiovascular disease.

Along with a balanced eating plan, exercise can foster a healthier body weight. The good news about exercise is that you reap heart-health benefits no matter what you weigh. See chapter 9 for the details on exercise, and how to make regular physical activity a part of your life.

Sufficient sleep. Sleep is often the first thing to go when life gets busy, hot flashes hit, or you feel stressed. Regular sleep deprivation can make you cranky, interfere with concentration and alertness, and may affect your relationships at work and home, your safety, and the safety of others. Inadequate sleep also deprives the body of the chance to heal and repair your heart and blood vessels, and increases the risk for obesity, high blood pressure, diabetes, and other health problems.

Sleep patterns evolve at midlife, and menopause and other bodily changes can make it more difficult to get restful, rejuvenating sleep. Adults should sleep at least seven and probably no more than nine hours a night.[21]

Starting in perimenopause, you may experience more trouble falling asleep, staying asleep, and sleeping deeply enough, in part because of hot flashes. One study found that perimenopausal women were most likely to sleep fewer than seven hours a night compared to postmenopausal women. In contrast, postmenopausal women were most likely to have poor-quality sleep.[22, 23]

Sleep disorders, such as insomnia and sleep apnea, can also interfere with a good night's sleep. During sleep apnea, people have many short pauses in breathing that keep them from sleeping deeply. Left untreated, sleep apnea can result in high blood pressure, stroke, and memory loss. Feeling sleepy during the day and being told you are snoring loudly at night could be signs of sleep apnea. If you suspect you have sleep apnea, consult a doctor who specializes in sleep problems.[24]

People with insomnia have trouble falling asleep, staying asleep, or both, which may leave them feeling like they haven't slept at all. Insomnia affects women more often than men, and older adults more than younger adults. Travel, work schedules that disrupt your sleep routine, depression, anxiety, and post-traumatic stress disorder (PTSD) can cause insomnia, as can certain over-the-counter and prescription drugs.[25]

In many cases, treating the underlying cause of insomnia may solve sleep problems; however, trouble sleeping can persist because of habits you formed to deal with a lack of sleep, including napping and worrying about sleep. Consider cognitive-behavioral therapy (CBT) to reduce stress and anxiety, which are often to blame for sleep problems.

Try these tactics to improve your slumber:

- Follow a regular sleep schedule. Go to sleep and get up at the same time each day, including on weekends, to work better with your body's natural rhythms.
- Avoid napping in the late afternoon or evening, as it may interfere with nighttime sleep. If you must nap, keep it to 20 minutes or less.
- Keep your bedroom at a comfortable temperature and as quiet as possible.

What Works for Us

Caring for others can be a drag on your sleep. It can be difficult to wind down after a long day of looking after children, a sick spouse, or elderly parents. During the three years my mom was ill, I developed a bedtime routine that worked for me: watch Netflix until my eyes closed. It was effective at the time because I needed a no-brainer escape from stress, but experts say to avoid screens to make it easier to fall asleep. Eventually, the stress subsided and I found screen time more stimulating than soothing. Now I read fiction before bed.

—Liz

- Stay physically active. Moderate and vigorous exercise on a regular basis can reduce the time it takes to get to sleep and help you to sleep more deeply, for longer. People with insomnia and obstructive sleep apnea may improve their sleep with physical activity.[26]
- Avoid going to bed with a very full stomach, and don't drink too much fluid before bed, either, including alcohol. Alcohol is relaxing at first, but it disrupts sleep later on in the night.
- Limit caffeine, especially later in the day. Caffeine is a stimulant that can keep you awake.
- Discuss all over-the-counter medications, prescription drugs, and dietary supplements you take with your doctor, nurse practitioner, or pharmacist to see if they may be interfering with sleep.
- Avoid nicotine. Nicotine is a stimulant that can affect sleep.

What Works for Us

If I wake up at night, I often start thinking of things I need to deal with the next day. As a way to "unload" so I can get back to sleep, I put a small notebook and a pen in my nightstand to write down what's on my mind so I can forget it for now. Sometimes I can barely read my writing in the morning, but it works!

—Hillary

How Diet Affects Heart Health

There's no doubt about the connection between food and heart health. While you eat food, not nutrients, it's important to know what food substances can harm the heart and which ones help it.

THE FACTS ABOUT FAT

Fat provides energy and makes food taste good. You also need fat for the essential fatty acids (EFAs)—linoleic acid and alpha-linolenic acid—it provides. In addition, fat helps the body absorb vitamins A, D, E, and K from foods and supplements and ferries them around the body.

Fat falls into three major categories: saturated, monounsaturated, and polyunsaturated. The majority of another type of fat in food, called trans fat, is mostly manufactured. All fats supply 9 calories per gram.

Foods typically contain a mixture of fat types, which are listed on the Nutrition Facts panel of packaged food products. All foods

Risk Factors for Heart Disease You Can't Control

Preventing heart disease is not completely up to you. There are some unavoidable contributors to heart health, including family history and your health history. While uncontrollable, these risk factors are important to keep in mind going forward.

- Having a father or brother who experienced a heart attack before age 55, or a mom or sister who had one before age 65.
- A history of being treated with certain chemotherapy drugs and radiation therapies.
- High blood pressure during pregnancy, which can result in high blood pressure in women years after delivery.
- Gestational diabetes, which increases the risk for type 2 diabetes later on.
- Women with polycystic ovary syndrome (PCOS) or endometriosis may have a greater risk for heart problems.

contain saturated, monounsaturated, and polyunsaturated fat, but one type of fat always prevails and tends to be associated with that food. For example, butter contains mostly saturated fat, and it is grouped with other foods with high saturated fat content, such as fatty meat and cheese. Olive oil contains mostly monounsaturated fat, and the primary type of fat in fish is polyunsaturated.

UNSATURATED FATS

Unsaturated fats are heart-healthy and should constitute the majority of the fat you eat. There are two types of unsaturated fats: monounsaturated and polyunsaturated.

Monounsaturated fat is the primary fat in olive oil, canola oil, avocados, almonds, pistachios, pecans, and peanuts. Foods such as soybean oil, corn oil, safflower oil, sunflower seeds, flaxseed, walnuts, and seafood contain the most polyunsaturated fat.

OMEGA-3 FATS

Omega-3 fats are a category of polyunsaturated fats that are beneficial for the heart as well as the brain. Alpha-linolenic acid (ALA), eicosapentaenoic acid (EPA), and docosahexaenoic acid (DHA) are the three main omega-3 fats. As a group, omega-3s lower blood triglyceride levels, slow the growth of plaque in arteries, and have a slight effect on lowering blood pressure. They also decrease the risk for arrhythmia (abnormal heartbeat), which can cause stroke and sudden death.[27]

ALA is an essential fatty acid, which means your body can't make it and you must get it from food. Flaxseed, flaxseed oil, walnuts, chia seeds, soy foods, and canola and soybean oils supply ALA. The body converts ALA to EPA and DHA, but at very low rates.[28] Seafood is the best natural source of DHA and EPA, and some foods, such as certain brands of milk, eggs, and yogurt, have added DHA. Consuming the suggested 8 ounces per week of a variety of seafood provides about 250 milligrams (mg) a day of EPA and DHA combined and is associated with better cardiac health, although studies suggest women consume far less than the recommended amounts.[29, 30] If you have heart disease or high triglycerides, ask your doctor if larger doses of omega-3 supplements may help and are safe for you. See chapter 10 for more on omega-3 supplements.

> ## What Works for Us
>
> ⟶⟵
>
> It can be tough to include seafood twice a week, even for the most motivated eater. Canned or pouched tuna fish and salmon and frozen shrimp save the day when time is tight. I use tuna and salmon in sandwiches and salads, and shrimp in stir-fries and pasta dishes. Done!
>
> —Liz

SATURATED FAT

For many people, eating excess saturated fat contributes to elevated LDL levels, which promote plaque build-up in arteries. While it's not necessary to completely avoid foods with saturated fat, you may need to curb your intake. Fatty meats, full-fat dairy foods, butter, lard, palm oil, palm kernel oil, and coconut oil contain high levels of saturated fat.

The American Heart Association (AHA) recommends no more than 6% of total daily calories from saturated fat. That means people eating about 2,000 calories a day should limit saturated fat intake to 120 calories daily, which translates to 13 grams a day. As part of a balanced eating plan, replacing saturated fat with polyunsaturated fat or monounsaturated fat reduces cardiovascular disease risk. Don't swap saturated fat calories for calories from refined grains like pasta, crackers, and fat-free sugary desserts, however. Research shows that does little to reduce heart disease risk.[31]

Trans fat is a type of fat that raises LDL cholesterol, lowers

HDL cholesterol, and is associated with a higher risk for type 2 diabetes. Though there are minute amounts of trans fat found naturally in fatty meats and full-fat dairy, it's been banned from highly processed foods produced in the United States.

CHOLESTEROL

Cholesterol is found only in animal foods. In a joint statement in 2013, the AHA and the American College of Cardiology said there was not enough strong scientific evidence to show that limiting dietary cholesterol lowers LDL cholesterol in the bloodstream.[32] However, it's important to note that some foods rich in cholesterol, such as fatty meats and full-fat dairy foods, are also high in saturated fat and should be limited for that reason.

OTHER FACTS ABOUT DIET

Fat isn't the only thing you should be monitoring. Several other nutrients play a role in heart health:

Fiber. Fiber, found only in plant foods, protects against heart disease as part of a balanced eating plan. Observational studies of large groups of people suggest that consuming higher amounts of fiber is linked to a lower risk for heart disease, stroke, and diabetes. There are two types of dietary fiber that support heart health in different ways.[33]

Soluble fiber dissolves in water and promotes lower levels of cholesterol and glucose in the blood. Foods rich in soluble fiber include oats, nuts, apples, berries, citrus fruit, pears, and legumes, such as black beans and lentils. Insoluble fiber does not dissolve in water and helps keep you fuller for longer, which aids weight control. Like soluble fiber, it also lowers blood glucose, and it prevents constipation and diverticulitis, an inflammation of the intestine. Wheat products, such as whole-wheat bread, cereal, and pasta, as well as brown rice, legumes, and vegetables, supply insoluble fiber.

Sodium. Sodium helps maintain normal fluid balance for healthy blood pressure and is also necessary for normal muscle contraction and nerve function. Research has found a connection between the amount of sodium you consume and the likelihood of high blood pressure and cardiovascular disease. Experts recommend limiting daily sodium intake to 2,300 milligrams to lower the risk for cardiovascular disease in healthy adults.[34]

Sodium is present in an array of forms in processed foods. You don't need to completely avoid sodium, but you may need to cut down on your intake. Packaged foods, restaurant fare, takeout, and convenience food items like canned soups and frozen dinners typically have more sodium than homemade versions. Fresh and lightly processed foods, such as fruit and vegetables, have the least sodium.

FOOD TYPE	AMOUNT OF SODIUM (MG)
Salt (1 teaspoon)	2,300
Grilled chicken sandwich, fast-food	1,237
Soy sauce (1 tablespoon)	1,024
Pizza, frozen (4 ounces)	890
Soup, canned (1 cup)	700–1,200
Vegetable juice, canned (8 ounces)	653

FOOD TYPE	AMOUNT OF SODIUM (MG)
Cottage cheese (1 cup)	390
Cottage cheese, no salt added (1 cup)	55

Source: U.S. Department of Agriculture, Agricultural Research Service, U.S.D.A. Food Composition Databases; available at https://ndb.nal .usda.gov/ndb/.

Pump up the Flavor

Most of the sodium we consume comes from packaged and restaurant foods. Choosing foods with less sodium allows you to better control sodium intake when cooking at home.

- Choose the freshest, most flavorful foods possible when cooking or eating out.
- Check food labels for sodium content.
- Opt for no-salt-added products.
- Add flavor with garlic, onions, herbs, and spices; lime, lemon, or orange juice; and vinegar or hot sauce.
- Roast vegetables without salt to bring out their natural flavors.
- Use monosodium glutamate (MSG), a source of umami, to reduce sodium intake. Umami is considered the fifth basic taste in addition to sweet, sour, salty, and bitter. MSG contains one-third of the sodium of salt and can be used in recipes and at the table.[35]

Potassium. Potassium works with sodium to normalize blood pressure, and it plays an essential role in nerve cell function and in proper muscle contraction. Potassium is also good for your bones. Experts suggest healthy women over the age of 19 consume 2,600 milligrams of potassium daily.[36] Certain medications to help manage blood pressure and type 2 diabetes may affect the potassium levels in the body. Talk with your doctor, nurse practitioner, or pharmacist about all the medications you take.

Fresh and lightly processed foods from all the food groups supply potassium. A balanced, plant-based eating plan can help you get the potassium your body needs to support your heart, and the rest of your body, too.

FOOD TYPE	AMOUNT OF POTASSIUM (MG)
Potato, medium, with skin, baked	941
White beans, canned, drained (½ cup)	595
Butternut squash, cubed (1 cup), cooked	582
Yogurt, plain, fat-free (1 cup)	579
Sweet potato, medium, with skin, baked	542
Salmon, Atlantic, wild (3 ounces), cooked	534
Orange juice, fresh (8 ounces)	496
Broccoli, chopped (1 cup), cooked	458

FOOD TYPE	AMOUNT OF POTASSIUM (MG)
Soybeans, mature (½ cup), cooked	443
Banana, 1 medium	422

Source: U.S. Department of Agriculture, Agricultural Research Service, U.S.D.A. Food Composition Databases; available at https://ndb.nal.usda.gov/ndb/.

Magnesium. Magnesium helps promote normal blood pressure and keeps your heart rhythm steady. It supports the immune system, regulates muscle and nerve function, and is involved in bone health. People with type 2 diabetes and celiac disease may have insufficient magnesium levels in their bodies. Eating plant foods that contain greater amounts of magnesium is associated with a lower risk for type 2 diabetes.[37] It can be difficult to get the suggested amount of magnesium, which is 320 milligrams daily for women over the age of 30. Generally speaking, foods with fiber also supply magnesium. Read more about how to include enough magnesium in your diet in chapter 7.

Calcium. Calcium is best known for building and maintaining strong bones and teeth, but the small amount of calcium circulating in the bloodstream is vital for blood pressure control and a regular heartbeat, among other functions. The suggested daily intake for calcium increases from 1,000 milligrams/day at age 50 to 1,200 milligrams/day after age 50. Dairy foods are naturally rich in calcium, and plant foods also provide calcium.

If you avoid dairy foods or eat them sparingly, consider adding more calcium-fortified foods to your eating plan. If that's not possible, you may need calcium supplements. Despite earlier concerns, researchers have concluded that there is no direct connection between taking calcium supplements and heart disease. Don't consume more than 2,500 milligrams of calcium on a daily basis, however.[38]

The beauty of the Menopause Diet Plan is that it is rich in fiber, healthy fats, potassium, calcium, and magnesium, and low in saturated fat and cholesterol. It's a delicious way to eat for heart health and overall well-being.

4

DIALING BACK
DIABETES RISK

Diabetes runs in my family and I am doing everything
possible to avoid it.

—Meg, age 53

Menopause paves the way for an increased risk of a number
of health problems including diabetes, that, if not proactively managed, can cast serious shade in this phase of
life and beyond. A constellation of conditions that involve abnor-
malities in blood sugar, or glucose, levels collectively increase a
woman's risk of developing type 2 diabetes, which unfortunately
is so common it sometimes feels like we throw this term around
without fully appreciating the catastrophic effect it can exert on
quality of life.

According to the Centers for Disease Control and Prevention
(CDC), about 17% of U.S. adults ages 45 to 64 have diabetes,
and almost 41% of people in that age bracket have prediabetes.[1]
Among all women over age 18, about 12% have diabetes and 31%
have prediabetes. That's one in eight women with diabetes and one
in three with prediabetes, and many of them don't know they have
the conditions.[2] Although the rate of diabetes increases with age
for both men and women, research suggests it may be higher in

women in their 60s and beyond.[3] Women who experience menopause before age 45 may be at higher risk for diabetes.[4]

Diabetes: A Simple Explanation

Diabetes is a chronic disease whereby the body has a reduced ability to clear glucose out of the blood and into the cells after eating
or drinking anything that contains carbohydrates, leading to high
blood glucose. Type 2 diabetes, the most common type, is caused
by the coexistence over time of two conditions: insulin resistance
(IR) and chronic inflammation. This results in a progressive state
in which the body needs to produce higher than normal amounts
of insulin to clear glucose out of the blood after a meal or snack. IR
occurs on a spectrum: It starts at a low level, where there's no easy
test to see that it's happening; as it progresses, IR eventually shows
up as prediabetes, and if not addressed through diet and lifestyle,
may progress to diabetes. You can inherit an increased risk of diabetes, yet having no known relatives with diabetes does not mean
you're without risk.

According to the CDC, diabetes is the seventh leading cause of
death in women in the United States, but since diabetes increases
the risk of four of the six causes of death preceding it, many experts believe its effect on life expectancy is much greater.[5] Diabetes
is associated with a host of other health problems, including heart
disease, stroke, amputations, kidney failure, cancer, and cognitive
(brain function) problems. Type 2 diabetes is linked to a 50% increased risk of dementia, and a recent analysis of studies involving
over 1.7 million people found the risk of Alzheimer's disease is
higher in people with diabetes.[6] Research tells us that the risk of all
these problems can be greatly reduced, or even avoided altogether,

when healthy lifestyle changes are implemented early on. As the old saying goes, an ounce of prevention is worth a pound of cure!

Diabetes Prevention from the Inside Out

For a better understanding of diabetes, let's dive deeper into what's involved in maintaining normal blood glucose levels, and what can go wrong.

The term *diabetes* is a catchall that covers a number of metabolic conditions involving high blood glucose. These include type 1 diabetes, type 2 diabetes, prediabetes, and gestational diabetes.

Regulating blood glucose levels requires an assist from insulin, a hormone produced by the pancreas. In type 1 diabetes, accounting for only about 10% of cases, the cells that make insulin are destroyed due to an autoimmune problem. Ninety percent of people with diabetes have type 2, caused by a progressive loss of insulin function due to IR, where the cells are insensitive to insulin's action. Prediabetes is exactly what it sounds like—a serious red flag for diabetes risk. An estimated 70% of people with prediabetes will eventually develop type 2 diabetes if prediabetes is not addressed with diet and lifestyle changes, and with medication, if necessary.[7] Gestational diabetes is also caused by IR, and any woman who had it during pregnancy is at increased risk of type 2 diabetes later in life, and even more so if she gains weight with age. Glucose intolerance can also sometimes be caused by medications, the most common being steroids like prednisone.

Several metabolic changes that occur during the peri- and menopausal years can increase diabetes risk, including an increase in belly fat, a slowing metabolism, impaired insulin secretion, and less sensitivity to the action of insulin. Whether menopause itself increases the risk of diabetes independent of aging is unclear.[8]

As mentioned, most cases of diabetes are caused by IR. Type 2 diabetes is IR in its most advanced form, but everyone with type 2 diabetes had prediabetes. And anyone with prediabetes had a period of time preceding it when they had IR, but their body was able to compensate by secreting more insulin, and glucose levels remained normal. However, the extra effort to produce insulin can eventually exhaust the pancreas, reducing insulin production and leading to full-blown type 2 diabetes. Unfortunately, there are no good tests for that "pre-prediabetes" phase, but there are risk factors that are red flags for IR:

- Being overweight
- Age 45 years or older
- Having a parent or sibling with type 2 diabetes
- Being physically active fewer than three times a week
- Having a history of gestational diabetes or giving birth to a baby who weighed more than 9 pounds
- Being of African American, Hispanic/Latino American, American Indian, or Alaska Native decent (some Pacific Islanders and Asian Americans are also at higher risk)[9]

Ground zero for reducing diabetes is managing IR—ideally, way before it affects glucose tests—and it's important to grasp what's happening with IR and how you can influence it.

Understanding Insulin

To understand IR and how to reverse it, you must appreciate how insulin works under healthy conditions. Insulin is one of a number of energy-storing growth hormones released into the blood after we eat that tells the nutrients where to go and what to do after digestion. Insulin is involved in the metabolism of protein and fat, but its major action is to clear the glucose created from eating carbohydrates out of the blood and direct it into the cells to be used as fuel. Insulin is produced by the pancreas, which detects how much glucose is in your blood after eating and releases what it thinks is enough insulin to lower glucose levels to normal. Insulin then circulates in the body like millions of little keys, efficiently unlocking cells to allow glucose to enter by connecting with one of many "keyholes" on the surface of the cell called insulin receptors. Within about two to three hours of eating, much of insulin's work is done, and glucose and insulin levels return to normal.

Generally speaking, insulin's job is to keep blood glucose levels roughly in the 70 to 115 milligrams per deciliter (mg/dl) range throughout the day. If glucose levels dip low, this is called *hypoglycemia*, which can leave you feeling "fuzzy" and hungry, often craving the carbohydrates the body relies on to replenish its blood glucose supply. High blood glucose, or *hyperglycemia*, happens when the body is unable to properly regulate glucose levels, the severity of which dictates whether you have prediabetes or diabetes. Unless blood glucose levels are very high or very low, there are generally no symptoms, so periodic screening for prediabetes and diabetes is key.

As you can see, in its role as a facilitator of energy processing, normal insulin action is critical to human survival. Unfortunately, in recent decades insulin's actions have morphed from being life-saving to potentially life-threatening as our modern world has progressively collided with our primitive biology. Scientists call this a "genetic mismatch," whereby genetic tendencies that were helpful become harmful under the conditions of modern life.

Insulin Resistance:
From Helpful to Harmful

Throughout history, starvation has been a major threat to human survival, so evolution has honed our metabolism to efficiently use nutrients when they're available and to hoard whatever's left over.

After we've eaten, insulin's primary task is to sweep glucose into the cells to be used as fuel, but its job description as a growth hormone doesn't end there. Because our cells will only take on the glucose they can use immediately, insulin directs some of the glucose that must be cleared from the blood to a storage form called glycogen, where it can be called on for fuel at a later time. But glycogen also has a limited capacity to take on glucose, so to avoid waste, insulin converts any remaining excess glucose into triglycerides, or fat, which circulate in the blood and are also stored as body fat. During the menopausal transition, the preferred storage place for triglycerides is the belly, a pretty universal source of misery for women.

All this calorie storing was super-helpful to our cave-woman ancestors because the risk of starvation was real. But in the modern world, this same ability to stockpile fuel can backfire, causing too much body fat to accumulate for a famine that never comes. In a further cruel twist of nature, excess belly fat chugs out hormones and other substances, causing inflammation that further worsens IR.

You might be wondering why nature thought IR was ever a good idea. In a nutshell, under conditions of physiologic stress, such as starvation, IR aided survival by triggering a "stress response" to make sure the central nervous system (brain and nerves) got the glucose it needed. Without glucose, the central nervous system wouldn't survive. Muscles use most of the glucose, and IR benefited the body during food shortages. IR makes muscle cells resistant to the action of insulin which keeps more glucose circulating in the bloodstream for the central nervous system to use. Once the famine eventually ended, our ancestors' metabolisms returned to normal, making the excess fat and accompanying inflammation temporary.

Unfortunately, much about modern life is feeding into our primitive stress response, making something designed to be temporary more permanent. Excess calorie intake, sedentary lifestyles, and eating patterns with too many highly processed foods and not enough fruits, vegetable, whole grains, legumes, nuts, seeds, and seafood increase excess belly fat and inflammation, raising the risk of not just diabetes but also other pro-inflammatory conditions like cardiovascular disease and cancer.

To summarize, excess body fat and an unhealthy diet can encourage IR, which makes our pancreas work overtime to regulate blood glucose levels. Insulin secretion matches the volume of food eaten, so large meals mean more work for a pancreas that wasn't designed to handle giant sugary sodas and portions of food that significantly exceed our needs. This additional work over time can exhaust the pancreas so that it is no longer able to secrete enough insulin, resulting in progressively higher blood levels. The good news is that right up to the threshold of diabetes, IR can be reversed, and the earlier you address it, the better.

Non-alcoholic Fatty Liver Disease: A Scary Consequence of Insulin Resistance

Belly fat not only worsens IR and heightens risk of diabetes, it also raises the risk of an increasingly common condition called non-alcoholic fatty liver disease, or NAFLD. NAFLD is the most common cause of chronic liver disease in the Western world that isn't related to alcohol and is currently estimated to affect 25% of adults in the United States. This number is expected to increase, with NAFLD estimated to eventually become the number one cause of liver failure requiring transplant. One study of postmenopausal women found that almost 40% had NAFLD based on abdominal ultrasounds. Fortunately, NAFLD responds positively to changes in diet and lifestyle habits like those outlined in this book, including losing 7 to 10% of your body weight.[10]

Know Your Numbers

There are three different ways to determine blood glucose levels: a fasting plasma glucose test (FPG), a hemoglobin A1C test (sometimes called glycosylated hemoglobin), and an oral glucose tolerance test (OGTT).[11] These tests determine whether you have normal glucose metabolism, prediabetes, or diabetes. It's important to be retested periodically, as the risk of diabetes increases with age. These blood tests should be conducted in a health-care setting (not with your friend's home glucose monitoring kit!).

The following is a description of the standard tests for prediabetes and diabetes.

FASTING PLASMA GLUCOSE TEST

This test requires you to fast overnight for eight to ten hours before your blood is drawn. A normal fasting plasma glucose is less than 100 milligrams per deciliter (mg/dl); 100 to 125 mg/dl is considered prediabetes, and 126 mg/dl or higher signals diabetes.

HEMOGLOBIN A1C

Sugar is "sticky," so a certain amount of it will cling to the hemoglobin cells in your blood. Hemoglobin cells live for approximately three months, so the hemoglobin A1C test result is considered a reflection of your average blood glucose levels within this time frame. A level of 5.6% or less is considered normal, 5.7 to 6.4% is considered prediabetes, and greater than or equal to 6.5% is considered diabetes.

ORAL GLUCOSE TOLERANCE TEST

This test is used less often and requires an overnight fast. Your blood glucose is checked in the morning after fasting, and again two hours later after drinking a concentrated glucose solution that contains 75 grams of glucose (the equivalent of drinking 23 ounces of sugary soda very quickly). A normal blood glucose level two hours after the glucose drink is less than 140 mg/dl, 140 to 199 mg/dl is considered prediabetes, and equal to or greater than 200 mg/dl is considered diabetes.

Testing for prediabetes is simple and noninvasive and can easily be rolled into an annual physical. If you have any of the risk factors for prediabetes listed here, please see the writing on the wall and start making changes instead of waiting until you are flunking your glucose tests. Intervening in the "pre-prediabetes" phase is the best defense against developing diabetes.

SCREENING FOR PREDIABETES AND DIABETES

According to the American Diabetes Association (ADA), certain groups of people should be tested and subsequently screened for prediabetes on a regular basis. Screening should begin at age 45, or sooner in all adults who are overweight (BMI of 25 or greater) and have additional risk factors, including:

- Physical inactivity
- First-degree relatives with diabetes
- High-risk race or ethnicity (African American, Latino, Native American, Asian American, Pacific Islander)
- Hypertension (greater than 140/90 millimeters of mercury [mmHg] or on medication for hypertension)
- HDL cholesterol level of less than 35 mg/dl and/or triglyceride level of greater than 250 mg/dl
- Women with polycystic ovary syndrome
- History of cardiovascular disease

Conditions that Strongly Suggest Insulin Resistance

There are two common conditions in which IR is known to be a major player: metabolic syndrome and polycystic ovary syndrome (PCOS). Being diagnosed with either strongly suggests underlying IR, and both are considered major risk factors for the development of diabetes. Let's learn a bit more about each condition.

METABOLIC SYNDROME

This incidence of metabolic syndrome is skyrocketing, contributing to the epidemic of diabetes and heart disease in a major way. According to the National Cholesterol Education Program, 44% of the U.S. population over age 50 meet the criteria for metabolic syndrome, as do 87% of people with diabetes.[12] Like type 2 diabetes, metabolic syndrome is driven by IR and chronic inflammation, and is characterized by a collection of cardiovascular risk factors.[13] Risk of metabolic syndrome increases with age, so it's an important health risk to consider through the menopausal years.

Metabolic syndrome is diagnosed when three or more of the following measurements are present:

- Abdominal obesity (excessive belly fat)
- Triglyceride level of 150 milligrams per deciliter (mg/dl) or greater
- HDL cholesterol level of less than 40 mg/dl in men or less than 50 mg/dl in women
- Blood pressure of 130/85 millimeters of mercury (mmHg) or higher
- Fasting glucose of 100 mg/dl or greater[14]

Although this may vary by race, excess belly fat is generally defined as a waist circumference of 40 inches (102 centimeters) or more for men and 35 inches (88 centimeters) or more for women. People with metabolic syndrome also have a tendency for their blood to clot more easily and are more likely to have chronic inflammation in their bodies (which can be diagnosed with a C-reactive protein test, a marker for inflammation in the blood).[15] Although any of these factors can increase your risk for heart attack—and individually each risk factor should be aggressively treated—when present together, as in metabolic syndrome, the risk of having cardiovascular problems is significantly greater. A review of the research on metabolic syndrome found it doubled the risk of cardiovascular disease, heart attack, and stroke and increased the chance of dying from any cause by 50%.[16] Other risk factors for metabolic syndrome include already having diabetes, having a parent or sibling with diabetes, or having PCOS. If you take medication to control one or more of the factors for metabolic syndrome, including triglycerides, glucose, or blood pressure, and your levels are normal, it's still considered a risk factor.

POLYCYSTIC OVARY SYNDROME

Polycystic ovary syndrome affects 5 to 10% (possibly more) of all women, and is the main cause of infertility related to irregular or absent ovulation. PCOS has been recognized as being a major risk factor for prediabetes, diabetes, and heart disease. Like metabolic syndrome, PCOS is a complex problem, but it is believed that IR is a significant player in at least 75% of cases. Insulin is a hormone, and as such has the ability to interfere with the exquisite hormonal balance needed to trigger ovulation, leading to trouble conceiving. Women with PCOS also often produce excess levels of testosterone that cause abnormal hair growth on the face and other areas on the body, hair loss on the crown of the head, and acne.

Research suggests more than 50% of women with PCOS will have diabetes or prediabetes before the age of 40.[17] Although PCOS is often associated with reproductive problems, as a genetic condition it sticks around after menopause, increasing diabetes risk for life. You can read more about the diet and lifestyle management of PCOS in *The PCOS Diet Plan: A Natural Approach to Health for Women with Polycystic Ovary Syndrome*.[18]

There are no universal signs and symptoms of IR, but in our experience many people who have IR report similar complaints that may be related, including the following:

- Fluctuations in energy level throughout the day
- Frequent hunger, and after eating not feeling full for long
- Binge eating at meals
- Constant cravings for sweets and other refined (white) carbohydrates, like white bread, crackers, pasta, or sweets
- Irritability if going too long without eating, which might not be long at all compared to people without IR
- Severe intolerance to low-calorie diets, particularly those that severely limit carbohydrates

Clearly you can experience these symptoms for a variety of reasons, but if this sounds like you, they are worth paying attention to.

As scary as all this is, not all the news is bad. According to the CDC, there is evidence that progression to diabetes among those with prediabetes is *not* inevitable, and we've seen that in our own practices. Research from the highly respected Diabetes Prevention Program (DPP) study has shown that people with prediabetes who

lose at least 7% of their body weight and engage in moderate physical activity at least 150 minutes a week can prevent or delay diabetes, and even return their blood glucose levels to normal. This
study compared a diet and lifestyle intervention to treatment with
a common diabetes medication called metformin. After about
three years, compared to a no-intervention group, the people in
the metformin group were 31% less likely to have progressed on to
diabetes, while those in the intensive diet and lifestyle intervention
group were 58% less likely to have developed diabetes, making it
the most effective way to prevent or delay type 2 diabetes.[19]

Experts estimate that up to 89% of type 2 diabetes could be
prevented. Several factors influence how sensitively any individual
responds to insulin. Research by Gerald Reaven, M.D., the first
scientist to identify the risks associated with metabolic syndrome,
suggests about 25% of that variability is due to being overweight,
25% is related to fitness level, and the remaining 50% is genetic.[20]

There's plenty of room for reducing your risk for diabetes,
whether or not you have a genetic predisposition. Though some
people require medication, many of our patients reverse the symptoms of prediabetes and type 2 diabetes with a healthier eating
plan and regular exercise.

The Lowdown on Carbohydrates

Because carbohydrates affect blood glucose levels the most, it's un-
derstandable that you might conclude that eating carbs increases
your risk of diabetes, and that you should avoid or seriously limit
carbs to reduce your risk for type 2 diabetes. But that's not what
the science says. Studies have tied even some of the most demon-
ized carbohydrate-containing foods to *lower* rates of diabetes!

Carbohydrate-containing foods include fruits, vegetables (although most vegetables are very low in carbohydrates and have a minimal effect on blood glucose levels), grains, and legumes. Milk and yogurt also contain carbohydrates. Though cheese is made from milk, most of the carbohydrates don't survive fermentation, so aged cheese contains little to no carbohydrates. Healthy carbohydrate-rich foods provide many important nutrients that we miss out on if we over-restrict them, including dietary fiber. What matters is the quality and quantity of carbohydrates consumed.

Quality refers to the carbohydrates' nutritional contributions to your diet and whether your digestive tract needs to work a little harder to break these carbs down to glucose. For example, the complex carbohydrates in foods such as sweet potatoes, legumes, and whole-wheat bread take longer to digest. This extra work means a more gradual rise in blood glucose after eating, which is easier for your body to manage.

Then there are the more refined carbohydrates that have little to offer beyond calories, including sugary sodas, candy, cake, cookies, ice cream, chips, and other snack foods, which are low-quality. There's no denying their taste appeal and the strong emotional connection many of us have with these foods. But highly processed carbohydrate-rich foods are truly "foods for fun" that, if routinely eaten in excess, may harm your health.

Foods that contain highly processed carbohydrates provide few vitamins and minerals, little to no fiber, and are often sources of excess calories and unhealthy fats. Excess intake of added sugars has been directly linked to increased risk of obesity, diabetes, heart disease, and a host of other health problems. Far too many of us are loading up on carbohydrates that have been stripped of their health-promoting attributes, like refined grains, sweets, and other highly processed foods packed with added sugars, and we are under-consuming those with clear health benefits. Added sugars should make up no more than 10% of your daily calories, but about one in ten Americans gets 25% or more of his or her calories from added sugars, about one-third of which come from sugar-sweetened beverages.[21]

The quantity of carbs you eat ultimately dictates how high your blood glucose will go after eating. Besides lacking healthy nutrients, foods with refined carbohydrates are more easily digested; in a way, the carbohydrates have been predigested by processing, so your body has much less work to do to finish them off, making it easier for them to spike your blood glucose. Examples of this are refining brown rice to white rice, whole-wheat flour to white flour, and whole fruit to juice. It's not that these more refined examples provide no nutrition—juice retains its vitamins and other nutrients, and refined grains are fortified with iron and vitamins. However, refining depletes the fiber found in whole grains, fruits, and vegetables and reduces the phytonutrients—beneficial plant substances.

Whether a carbohydrate is whole foods–based or highly processed, small amounts of carbohydrates bump your blood glucose up a little, and large amounts bump it up a lot. Portion control requires hunger management, which is why it's so important to eat often enough over the day to avoid arriving at your next meal or snack starved and at high-risk for overeating.

The biggest consumers of glucose in the body are our muscles and central nervous system (brain, spinal cord, and nerves), which prefer a steady supply of fuel. Brain cells need twice as much energy as the other cells in the body, which accounts for the sensations of weakness, moodiness, trouble focusing, and in some people, actual shakiness when we go too long without eating. These symptoms can cause intense cravings for carbohydrates as the brain seeks to replenish its preferred source of fuel. Depending on taste preferences, the call may be for a sugary treat, something starchy like bread, or salty and crunchy like chips.

Balancing your food choices and taking proactive steps to manage your hunger can help you avoid relying heavily on willpower, which is supposed to prevent us from eating too much, but which we naturally possess very little of. Balance happens by pairing carbohydrates with proteins, healthy fats, and more veggies at meals to make it easier to forgo that extra portion of rice, potatoes, or pasta. This applies to snacks, too. Pairing carbohydrate with protein, like peanut butter or cheese and crackers, or fruit and a small handful of nuts, will help you feel fuller longer.

According to a recent analysis of forty-eight studies on dietary patterns and risk of diabetes, eating in a way consistent with the Mediterranean and other plant-based diets that include vegetables, fruits, legumes, poultry, and seafood is associated with significantly lower rates of diabetes. On the other hand, dietary patterns including a lot of red and processed meats, sugar-sweetened beverages, refined grains, high-fat dairy, and fried foods are linked to greater diabetes risk.[22] Our Menopause Diet Plan, outlined in detail in chapter 11, is in line with these findings.

The brain and other organs need fuel, and carbohydrates are the preferred source. By choosing foods with high-quality carbohydrates—whole fruits, vegetables, whole grains, legumes, milk, and yogurt—and spreading them out over the day in moderate quantities in balanced meals and snacks, your blood glucose levels will roll like gentle hills and valleys over the day rather than spiking and dropping, which is likely to happen when you go too long without eating and then overeat in response. That said, there is room for special treats in every eating plan once your other needs for healthful foods are met.

How Much Carbohydrate
Is "Not Too Much?"

The easiest way to estimate a reasonable amount of carbohydrate to aim for at a meal is to model the MDP plate (see page 207) or follow the meal plans in chapter 11.

How much total carbohydrate you should eat in a day varies based on calorie needs and level of physical activity, but remember that it's the quantity eaten per meal or snack that affects peak blood glucose levels. A moderate amount of carbohydrate hovers at 45 to 60 grams of carbohydrate per meal. Some sedentary women may feel they do fine with 30 grams of carbohydrate per meal, but our goal is for you to increase your physical activity, which may mean you will need more carbohydrates. A reasonable snack goal is 15 to 30 grams of carbohydrate. These numbers include only carbs from whole grains, starchy vegetables, fruit, milk, yogurt, and sweets (keep this in mind when looking at your food logging app, which will list every morsel of carbohydrate you've eaten). For example, according to the American Diabetes Association Exchange Lists for Meal Planning,[23] there's roughly 15 grams of carbohydrate in an average-size piece of fruit, ⅓ cup of cooked brown rice or quinoa, ½ cup of sweet potatoes, or a small container of plain Greek yogurt. Most vegetables, such as lettuce, green beans, and broccoli, are very low in carbohydrates, so for diabetes prevention they're considered "free." (It's safe to assume no one ever developed diabetes from eating too much broccoli!) Aiming for a general per meal and snack carbohydrate goal doesn't mean you sometimes won't eat more or less, but it provides a rough estimate for those interested in understanding the carbohydrate content of their favorite foods, reading nutrition labels, or interpreting the data derived from food logging apps.

What Works for Us

‑╼‑

I was raised in a family with two siblings with type 1 diabetes, so I credit my mom for the healthy eating habits she taught us growing up. Fortunately, I adopted a regular physical activity routine in college, which I'm especially grateful for now that I'm at an age where diabetes prevention is a priority.

—Hillary

Focus on Fiber

Your intestinal tract does much more than digest food and absorb nutrients. It is home to tiny bacteria that play a big role in your health. These microbes are not a part of you in the same way as your heart, brain, and kidneys are, yet they are just as important. Gut microbes need you and you need them. As host, you provide food, water, and warmth. In return, bacteria help you break down food your body cannot digest, produce B vitamins and vitamin K, reduce inflammation, and help keep your blood glucose levels in check.

The digestive system has its own nervous system, harbors cells that produce hormones and other compounds that direct bodily functions, regulates metabolism, and contains the largest concentration of immune cells found anywhere in the body. In short, the gut is a vital organ that's deeply involved in overall health, including blood glucose regulation and weight control, and it needs fiber.

For the most part, gut bacteria munch on fiber to fuel their activity. Fiber is a type of carbohydrate that the body cannot digest. When fiber reaches the colon, bacteria ferment it and produce compounds that benefit the gut and overall health.

There are many types of fiber in food, and while not all fibers feed gut microbes, they are all vital for good health. Experts recommend eating 30 grams of fiber daily or more. Use this list to help figure out fiber and check the Nutrition Facts panel on food labels for fiber content.

FIBER TYPES	AMOUNT OF FIBER (GRAMS)
Navy beans (½ cup), cooked	10
Lentils (½ cup), cooked	8
Black beans (½ cup), cooked	8
Garbanzo beans (½ cup), cooked	8
White beans (½ cup), cooked	6
Pear, 1 medium	6
Avocado (½ cup)	5
Soybeans (½ cup), cooked or roasted	5
Peas (½ cup), cooked	4
Chia seeds (1 tablespoon)	4
Apple, medium, with skin	4

FIBER TYPES	AMOUNT OF FIBER (GRAMS)
Raspberries (½ cup)	4
Potato, medium, with skin, baked	4
Sweet potato, medium, flesh only, baked	4
Almonds (1 ounce)	4
Oats, steel-cut (¼ cup), uncooked	4
Artichokes, quartered (½ cup), jarred	3
Barley (½ cup), cooked	3
Broccoli (½ cup), cooked	3
Orange, 1 medium	3
Banana, 1 medium	3
Quinoa (½ cup), cooked	3
Whole-wheat bread (1 slice)	3
Pistachios, shelled (1 ounce)	3
Asparagus (7 spears), cooked	2
Peanuts (1 ounce), roasted	2
Walnuts (1 ounce)	2
Tomato (½ cup), chopped	1

Source: U.S. Department of Agriculture, Agricultural Research Service, U.S.D.A. Food Composition Databases; available at https://ndb.nal.usda.gov/ndb/.

While nourishing gut bacteria, fiber also helps to head off constipation, which is having fewer than three bowel movements a week, having dry, hard stools, or straining to move your bowels and feeling like you may need to go again. Constipation affects women more than men and often gets worse after menopause, as declining estrogen may reduce the speed at which food travels through the intestinal tract.

In addition to consuming the recommended amounts of fiber and fluid to keep things moving along, exercise stimulates the gut to keep you more regular. Check with your doctor or nurse practitioner about the medications you take, as some, such as antidepressants and over-the-counter sleeping pills, may contribute to constipation. Depending on your situation, you may need powdered fiber supplements in addition to adequate fiber from foods. Ask your healthcare provider for advice about supplements, and if you need a laxative, and what type.

What Counts as Sugar

Any of the following terms indicate an added sugar:

Brown sugar	Honey
Corn sweetener	Invert sugar
Corn syrup	Lactose
Dextrose	Maltose
Fructose	Malt syrup
Fruit juice concentrates	Molasses
Glucose	Raw sugar
High-fructose corn syrup	Sucrose
	Sugar
	Syrup

What Works for Us

I *love* sugar. While I know that sugar doesn't cause dia-betes, I have taken steps to limit my added sugar intake, but I will only go so far. I've tried drinking coffee and tea without the sweet stuff, but it didn't work for me, and probably never will. However, choosing sugar-free cere-als and limiting baked goods has made a big dent in my added sugar intake.

—Liz

The Skinny on Non-nutritive Sweeteners

As concern about excessive sugar intake has increased, an ever-expanding list of non-nutritive sweeteners (NNS) has infiltrated the food supply. Those currently available include aspartame (Nutra-Sweet, Equal), saccharin (Sweet 'N Low, Sugar Twin), sucralose (Splenda), acesulfame-K (Sweet One, Sunett), and stevia (Truvia, Pure Via). NNSs are regulated by the U.S. Food and Drug Administration and are generally recognized as safe. One downside is that foods containing NNSs are generally highly processed and devoid of nutrients. Given the lack of consistent evidence showing benefits of consuming them, we suggest you play it safe and limit them to a serving a day, just in case scientists discover something harmful about them in the future.

Last but Definitely Not Least: Exercise for Diabetes Prevention and Management

Whether you love it, hate it, or fall somewhere in between, physical activity plays a critical role in diabetes prevention. Exercise acts as nature's insulin sensitizer by increasing the activity of glucose transporter 4 (GLUT 4), a protein in our cells that partners with insulin to shuttle glucose out of the blood and into muscle and fat cells.[24] Many studies confirm that exercise improves insulin sensitivity in people with prediabetes, whether or not they lose weight. In fact, in those with prediabetes, eating right and regular exercise may lower the risk of developing diabetes by an average of 50%![25] Ask anyone with diabetes who checks her blood glucose regularly and she'll testify to the blood glucose-lowering effects of exercise, including its ability to reduce the amount of medication needed to control the condition. Both aerobic and strengthening exercises offer diabetes-prevention benefits (muscles act as "glucose sponges" so the more the better!). Chapter 9 explains all the health-promoting effects of regular exercise, especially through the menopause transition and beyond.

5

HOW TO PROTECT
YOUR BRAIN

Between the hot flashes and getting up to pee, I don't
sleep very well and it's starting to affect my energy and
concentration.

—*Jane, age 51*

Though it weighs only about three pounds, the brain is Chief
Executive Officer of the body. As head boss, your brain con-
trols all your bodily functions and behavior, as well as the
way you think and feel. It's what makes you—you.

Once you're in your 40s, it may seem as if your brain has a
mind of its own. Perhaps you are more irritable than usual, have
hot flashes that interfere with sleep at night and thinking clearly
during the day, or can't always remember why you walked into a
room or where you put your keys.

Hormonal changes are likely to blame for the memory lapses,
moodiness, and fatigue that women experience during midlife. Declining estrogen levels, and aging in general, increase the chances
of chronic conditions that affect the brain in much the same way
as they affect the heart. For example, the risk for having a stroke
doubles in the decade after menopause.

There is a silver lining, though. Healthy lifestyle habits help take the edge off both the effects of estrogen loss and the influence of getting older. Are you seeing a pattern yet? In this chapter, we discuss how to stay sharp, feel energetic, and safeguard the brain, your most valuable asset.

Brain Fog: It's Real

Do you ever have trouble concentrating, multitasking, or coming up with a word? It happens to us all the time! So-called brain fog can be alarming for midlife women. The good news is that it's highly unlikely that dementia, including Alzheimer's disease, is the reason for changes in *cognitive function*, a term that encompasses memory, reasoning, and learning.

More often than not, perimenopause and menopause tinker with learning, mood, and memory, and may affect your ability to recall facts, figures, and memories. The hippocampus, the part of the brain that stores most memory, is particularly vulnerable to hormonal shifts.[1] In addition to hormonal dips, researchers have found perimenopausal and menopausal women are less efficient at processing glucose in the brain, which can hamper mental sharpness and energy levels because the brain requires a constant supply of glucose to perform at peak function.[2]

In one study, researchers followed more than 400 women for fourteen years, periodically testing their ability to process information and memory. They found that as levels of estradiol, the form of estrogen produced in the ovaries, dropped over the years, women did not perform as well on memory and learning tests. However, one-third of the postmenopausal women with low estradiol levels scored high on the tests and showed brain activity similar to that of premenopausal women. It may be that some women's brains resist the effects of declining estradiol, or it could be that healthy habits, including regular physical activity, protect the brain, or a combination of both.[3]

There is a light at the end of the menopause tunnel. Experts say that, for the most part, the postmenopausal brain adjusts to the availability of less estrogen (fat tissue produces estrogen, so you still have some). In a four-year study that involved more than 2,300 women, declines in memory and learning ability during the transition to menopause bounced back after menopause was complete.[4]

If you're out of sorts, consult your doctor or nurse practitioner. Health professionals typically check for thyroid disease, one or more vitamin deficiencies, and infections as reasons for mental fogginess, and those can be legitimate causes. However, it's likely that perimenopause and menopause are at the root of your cognitive symptoms, so discuss your menstrual history in detail with your healthcare provider.

The Effects of Stress on the Brain

Stress can mess with memory and other cognitive skills. The years leading up to menopause often coincide with a stage of life that's full of other transitions, too. You may be sending kids to college or still have teens at home (or both), caring for elderly parents, working full time, or all of the above!

Stress is unavoidable, and it's actually necessary. Stress is a biological response designed to defend against dangerous situations. When you feel stressed, your brain mobilizes the rest of your body to take action, triggering the release of two hormones, adrenaline and cortisol, to prime you to stay and fight or run away. For our ancient ancestors, the stressor might have been the threat of an animal attack. In the modern world, the stressors are different, but the body's response hasn't changed.

The body's reaction to stress is meant to be short-lived and not always in the "on" position as it is for many midlife women. Once the threat, real or imagined, has passed, adrenaline and cortisol levels return to normal. Prolonged stress is different, as it increases cells' exposure to adrenaline and cortisol, which can promote weight gain and affect the digestive system, cardiovascular system, and mental health. For example, cortisol supplies the body with energy to respond to stressful situations, and by that we mean literally running away from what you perceive as dangerous. That can be a good thing, but it has a downside. Cortisol may cause elevated blood glucose levels that last longer than they should, which in turn stresses the pancreas to produce more insulin.

Cortisol can also mess with memory. In a study of midlife women and men, researchers found that higher blood levels of cortisol were associated with a lower brain volume, which is important because brain volume is linked to memory. There was a stronger link between cortisol levels and memory issues in women than in men, who were each tested twice, once at baseline and again about seven and a half years later. The study does not prove that cortisol is responsible for cognitive decline, but it does suggest a link.[5]

Research from the Study of Women's Health Across the Nation (SWAN) Sleep Study found that chronic stress interferes with adequate sleep. Anyone who has ever laid awake in bed at night worrying about financial or relationship problems knows that all too well. Ongoing fatigue limits brain function, including memory recall, learning, and processing of facts.[6]

Life will never be totally stress-free, but you should try to manage stress as much as possible. Chronic stress can lead to behaviors with the potential to harm the brain, including smoking, excess alcohol intake, and "stress-eating" fatty and sugary foods, like ice cream, cookies, and chips, on a regular basis.

Tips to Manage Stress

We all differ in how we interpret stress, based on how our brains are wired and our past experiences. Stressors are highly individual. Figure out what triggers stress for you and how best to react to it. It won't always be possible to avoid your triggers, but you can improve your reaction to negative situations. Stress management techniques include the following:

- Adequate sleep
- Eating an enjoyable, balanced diet
- Limiting or avoiding alcohol
- Regular physical activity
- Taking time for yourself every day, even if it's just 15 to 30 minutes
- Relaxation techniques, such as meditation
- Nurturing positive relationships with friends and family
- Asking for help

Anxiety

It's normal to feel anxious before giving a presentation, making a big decision, or trying to get through the holidays while working a full-time job and running a household, but unrelenting stress can lead to anxiety. The strain of dealing with several stressors at once can leave you feeling uneasy on a regular basis and could suggest an anxiety disorder, which includes intense and uncontrollable feelings of fear, worry, and panic that don't disappear easily, and may worsen with time. Anxiety disorders can interfere with your personal life and job performance, and can keep you from doing things that your friends and family appear to do with ease, such as travel, maintain a career, and socialize.

Health conditions, including thyroid problems and an irregular heartbeat, may cause anxiety or make it worse. Whatever the case, if your worries are getting in the way of living life to the fullest, seek help. Anxiety disorders are often treated with medication or talk therapy, or a combination of both.[7]

A diet based on lean protein foods, whole grains, fruits, and vegetables, and low in added sugars and caffeine, may help ease anxiety. Eat balanced meals regularly throughout the day, as drops in blood glucose levels can cause you to feel jittery and worsen anxiety. Stay hydrated to help your brain and body feel at its best.

What Works for Us

I have a tendency to get anxious, especially when I have a lot of work to do. I can't always completely control my emotions, but I have developed some time-out tactics to take the edge off my feelings, including taking a short walk, calling a friend, napping for 20 minutes, having a cup of soothing hot tea, or watching a favorite show. Finding a quiet place to sit, close my eyes, and breathe deeply, even if just for a few minutes, always helps, too.

—Liz

Depression

Depression is a real illness, just like heart disease or cancer, and it's probably more common than you think, especially during the menopausal transition. An estimated one in six American adults will experience depression at some point. The symptoms of depression include feelings of emptiness, hopelessness, decreased energy or fatigue, loss of interest in activities that you enjoy, and a persistent sad or anxious mood that lasts for at least two weeks.[8]

Feelings of depression do not mean you are weak, flawed, or at fault for how you feel. Experts say depression is caused by a combination of genetic, biological, environmental, and psychological factors, including a family history (blood relative) of depression, experiencing traumatic or stressful events, and going through major life changes, such as menopause.[9] Research suggests that women may be particularly prone to depression during perimenopause and menopause.[10]

In addition to changes in hormone levels, discomfort from hot flashes, poor sleep, and upsetting life events, such as divorce, death of a spouse, or unemployment, increase the odds for depression, while strong social support during the menopause transition helps to decrease depression.[11]

Depression can interfere with your relationships and with normal daily activities like working, eating, and sleeping. It may also be hard to maintain lifestyle habits that support overall health, including eating well, getting regular exercise, not smoking, and avoiding excessive alcohol intake.

If you're feeling sad and hopeless, don't expect to "shake it off." Depression is treatable. Consult your healthcare provider to rule out the possibility that your feelings are the result of medications you're taking or a medical condition.[12]

Stroke

Stroke. Just the word strikes fear into the heart of anyone who has experienced one or who knows someone who has, and for good reason. A stroke can be debilitating and life-threatening.

A stroke, or "brain attack," occurs when blood flow is cut off to an area of brain tissue. Blood supplies the brain with oxygen, and a stroke results in brain cell death. An ischemic stroke, by far the most common kind, is caused by a blockage in a blood vessel in the brain or neck. Atherosclerosis is the major reason for ischemic stroke, and a loss of estrogen may heighten the risk. One study found that women who reach menopause before age 42 were at greater risk for ischemic stroke after age 60.[13]

Hemorrhagic strokes, which are far less common, result from leaky vessels that cause bleeding into the brain or spaces surrounding the brain. A hemorrhagic stroke also causes brain cell death.[14]

Call 911 immediately if you sense you or someone that you're with is having a stroke. Waiting to seek medical help can lead to irreversible damage. The signs and symptoms of a stroke can include one or more of the following:

Sudden numbness or weakness of the face, arm, or leg, especially on one side of the body

Sudden confusion, or trouble talking or understanding speech

Sudden trouble seeing in one or both eyes

Sudden trouble walking, dizziness, or loss of balance or coordination

Sudden severe headache with no known cause

Other danger signs that may occur include double vision, drowsiness, and nausea or vomiting.

TIA: More than Just a Mini-Stroke

TIA stands for *transient ischemic attack*, which people may refer to as a "mini-stroke." Yet, a TIA is anything but mini in importance. A TIA is a temporary blockage of blood flow to the brain that doesn't cause permanent damage. During a TIA, the body relies on its own clot-busting powers to break down a blockage. Unfortunately, about one in three people who have a TIA will eventually experience a stroke, with about half occurring within a year after the TIA. Though TIA symptoms may fully resolve within an hour, seek medical help immediately if you're experiencing one or more of these symptoms:[15]

- Weakness, numbness, or paralysis in your face, arm, or leg, typically on one side of the body
- Slurred speech
- Difficulty understanding what other people are saying
- Blindness in one or both eyes or double vision
- Dizziness or loss of balance or coordination
- Sudden, severe headache with no known cause

Stroke Risk Factors

What's bad for the heart is bad for the brain, and the risk factors for stroke are very similar to those for heart attack. Here are the ones you cannot change:[16]

- *Sex.* Women have more strokes than men because they live longer.
- *Age.* Stroke can occur at any age, but the likelihood increases after age 55.
- *Race.* Stroke is most common among African Americans, even in young and middle-aged adults. An important risk factor for African Americans is sickle cell disease, which can cause a narrowing of arteries and disrupt blood flow. Hispanic Americans also have a much higher stroke risk than Caucasians.

Up to 80% of strokes are preventable with healthier lifestyle choices, according to the American Stroke Association. Controlling risk factors as early in life as possible reduces the likelihood of stroke later on. Here is what you can modify to head off stroke:

- *High blood pressure.* Of all the risk factors for stroke, high blood pressure is the single most important one. High blood pressure contributes to clogged arteries and weakens artery walls.
- *Smoking.* Smoking is associated with twice the risk of ischemic stroke and four times the chance for hemorrhagic stroke. Smoking is linked to the build-up of plaque in the carotid artery, the main blood vessel in the neck that supplies blood to the brain, raises blood pressure, and makes your blood more likely to clot and create a blockage.[17]
- *Irregular heartbeat.* A common heart disorder known as atrial fibrillation (irregular heart beat), or "afib," may cause blood clots that can break loose and block vessels in the brain or leading to it. If you have atrial fibrillation, work closely with a cardiac specialist to manage it.

- *Elevated "bad" cholesterol.* Excess levels of low-density lipo-protein (LDL) cholesterol, considered "bad" because it contributes to clogged arteries, increase the risk of blocked blood flow to the brain.
- *Diabetes.* Diabetes causes destructive changes in all blood vessels, including those in the brain and leading to it, and may double the risk of stroke. See chapter 4 for more on how to reduce the risk of diabetes and best manage it.
- *Sedentary lifestyle.* Regular physical activity helps to manage blood pressure, stress, blood cholesterol, body weight, and blood glucose levels, all of which play a role in stroke risk. Chapter 9 discusses the benefits of exercise in detail.
- *Poor diet.* The "Western diet," which is excessive in saturated fat, added sugar, and sodium, and low in healthy fats, fiber, and phytonutrients, likely contributes to stroke risk. See "Eat to Be Kind to Your Mind" (page 98) for how diet supports brain health.

What Works for Us

My dad died from a stroke at a relatively young age, and now that I'm past menopause, I pay closer attention to my own stroke risk. I can't do anything about my menopausal status or my age, but I keep close tabs on my blood pressure, lipid levels, and diet, and get regular exercise to help reduce my stroke risk.

—Liz

How to Dodge Dementia

Though some cognitive decline is a normal part of aging, dementia is different. Dementia is the loss of thinking, remembering, reasoning, and behavioral abilities. You don't have dementia simply because you forgot why you walked into a room, you missed a dentist appointment, or you can't come up with a word every so often. While annoying, temporary memory lapses are different from dementia, which disrupts daily living and activities as it ravages memory, language skills, visual perception, problem solving, self-management, and the ability to focus and pay attention. Dementia may also result in personality changes.[18]

Dementia destroys neurons, the most prominent type of cell in the brain and the other parts of the central nervous system. Neurons are information messengers. All sensations, movements, thoughts, memories, and feelings are the result of signals that pass from one neuron to the next. Neurons are the longest-living cells in the body, but they are not invincible. Though everyone loses some neurons, people with dementia lose far more. Symptoms of dementia show up when neurons stop working, lose connections with other brain cells, and die in droves.

The causes of dementia vary. In Alzheimer's disease, the most common form of dementia in older adults, neurons are destroyed by certain compounds that accumulate in and around them. Alzheimer's targets neurons in the hippocampus, the part of the brain that stores memories, facts, and figures. As the disease progresses, the volume of the hippocampus declines, and the disease damages other areas that control language, reasoning, and behavior. Experts think that a smaller hippocampus may be a risk factor for Alzheimer's disease.[19]

In vascular dementia, the second most common form of dementia in older adults, stroke injures the blood vessels that supply the brain with oxygen-rich blood and other nutrients. The symptoms of vascular dementia can be similar to those of Alzheimer's, and both conditions may occur at the same time.

What Works for Us

There is a history of both ischemic and hemorrhagic stroke in my family, but smoking and uncontrolled diabetes and high blood pressure were likely at play in both instances. I try to focus on what I can control by eating well and being active almost daily, and I assume it will pay off. I'm super-focused on diabetes prevention as I have genes for that on both sides of the family.

—Hillary

Eat to Be Kind to Your Mind

There is no magic bullet to prevent dementia or cure Alzheimer's disease, which may run in families, but it's likely that diet and lifestyle choices slow the decline in cognitive skills. Large observational studies have associated eating patterns with less red and/or highly processed meats, added sugars, refined grains, and salt, and more fruits, vegetables, whole grains, nuts, legumes, and seafood with lower rates of dementia and age-related cognitive decline. The Mediterranean eating plan and the Dietary Approaches to Stop Hypertension (DASH) diet, described in chapter 1, are plant-based plans that help protect the heart and the brain in combination with other healthy lifestyle choices.

The Mediterranean–DASH Intervention for Neurodegenerative Delay (MIND) diet is a hybrid of the Mediterranean eating plan and DASH that may help prevent or slow brain degeneration. While the MIND diet is also plant-based, it makes specific suggestions for certain foods and food groups that are considered especially protective of brain health, including berries and green leafy vegetables, which contain high concentrations of anti-inflammatory compounds that guard against brain cell damage. The MIND diet also limits certain foods that may promote inflammation. For example, it recommends eating less than one serving a week each of red meat, cheese, fried or fast food, and pastries and sweets, and less than 1 tablespoon of butter a day.

Following the MIND diet has met with some success. An observational study of 923 people ages 58 to 98 years compared the effects of the MIND diet, the DASH diet, and the Mediterranean diet on the chances of developing Alzheimer's disease. The people in the study ate one of the three diets and were followed for an average of four and a half years. The researchers found that the groups who stuck very closely to any of the three diets reduced Alzheimer's disease risk, but that the MIND diet was particularly effective, even when people were only moderately compliant. Sticking closely to the MIND diet was associated with 53% less risk of Alzheimer's disease, while moderate adherence was linked to a 35% lower risk.[20] While the MIND diet fared better for reducing cognitive decline in this study, it's important to note that research suggests the Mediterranean way of eating is helpful, too. About 450 people, half of them women with a mean age of nearly 70 years, were asked to follow one of three eating patterns for six years:

- Mediterranean diet that included 1 liter (about 1 quart) of extra-virgin olive oil a week
- Mediterranean diet with 1 ounce mixed nuts per day
- A control diet, where participants received advice on reducing fat intake only

The groups that ate the Mediterranean diet with either olive oil or mixed nuts experienced significantly less cognitive decline than the group advised to lower fat intake.[21]

Another study showed that the DASH diet and exercise work better together to head off dementia. A clinical trial published in 2019 found that the duo improved memory in a group of 160 older people over age 55, who were physically inactive, and who had mild memory and thinking problems. When compared with a sedentary lifestyle, six months of moderate exercise plus a DASH eating plan boosted memory and thinking skills, including improvements in executive function, which is the ability to pay attention, get organized, complete tasks, and regulate behavior. Though the study was small, it was a clinical trial that proved the effects of diet and exercise on the brain.[22]

Even with a family history of cognitive function problems, a healthy diet, such as the Menopause Diet Plan, and regular exercise are helpful, according to an eight-year study published in 2019 that followed more than 196,000 people who were at least 60 years old. About half were women. The likelihood for dementia was cut by about half among those at high genetic risk when they closely adhered to a healthy lifestyle, which included not smoking, regular physical activity, healthy diet, and moderate alcohol consumption.[23]

Must-Have Nutrients for Brain Health

We talk a lot about the importance of dietary patterns for overall wellness, but we can't ignore certain nutrients that play a special role in brain health, including the following.

Omega-3 fats. As discussed in chapter 3, omega-3 fats are heart-healthy and support the brain much in the same way as they protect your ticker. Omega-3s are a vital part of the membranes that surround and protect each cell, which are particularly rich in DHA, one of the major omega-3s. Cells in the retina, the part of the eye that helps the brain interpret what you see, are also rich in DHA.

Seafood is a reliable source of DHA and EPA. Several observational studies have examined the effects of fish, EPA, and/or DHA intakes on cognitive function in healthy older adults. A reduction in the size of the hippocampus frequently appears before a person exhibits signs of Alzheimer's disease, and studies have tied higher omega-3 intake with larger brain and total hippocampus volumes, as well as improved cognitive test scores.[24, 25] A review of the results from twenty-one studies found that the greater the fish and dietary DHA intake, the lower the chances for dementia and Alzheimer's disease.[26]

As for mental health, a review article that assessed the outcomes of twenty-six studies involving more than 150,000 people found that higher fish intake was linked to a reduced risk of depression in both men and women.[27] Though the study didn't determine the type of fish or the amount that was most beneficial, the Dietary Guidelines for Americans advise adults to eat at least eight ounces of a variety of seafood weekly, in part for the omega-3 fats fish provides.[28]

Choline. Choline is part of every cell. Your body produces some choline, but doesn't make all that you need. That's why food, dietary supplements, or a combination, are essential to satisfy choline needs.

During pregnancy and early life, choline plays an important role in the development of the hippocampus—the brain's "memory center." The hippocampus is one of the only areas in the brain that produces cells into late adulthood, and some research shows an association between better cognitive performance and higher choline consumption in people without dementia. A study of 1,391 adults ages 36 to 83 showed that people with higher choline intakes had better verbal memory and visual memory as time progressed.[29] A review of the evidence about choline and brain health also suggests choline may preserve cognitive function, and an adequate supply of both choline and DHA may help to slow cognitive decline with aging and delay the development of Alzheimer's disease.[30]

Choline is found in a variety of foods, but it is concentrated in eggs, meat, poultry, seafood, and soy. For example, one large egg or ¾ cup roasted soybeans supply about 30% of your daily choline intake. Women of all ages need 425 milligrams of choline daily, but it appears most don't get enough. Data from the National Health and Nutrition Examination Survey (NHANES) shows that women consume an average of 278 milligrams of choline daily.[31] In addition, estrogen is necessary for the body to make choline, and research suggests that the choline needs of postmenopausal women are higher.[32]

So, you should be looking to supplement your diet if you limit or avoid animal foods. Most multivitamins don't contain much, if any, choline, and it's likely you'll need a separate choline pill. See chapter 10 for more about choline dietary supplements.

Vitamin B₁₂. Vitamin B_{12} supports the heart and the nervous system. It protects nerve cells and helps produce neurotransmitters that help nerve cells communicate. Experts estimate that up to 15% of the general population has a vitamin B_{12} deficiency; symptoms may include poor memory, confusion, depression, and dementia. Untreated vitamin B_{12} deficiency can result in irreversible nerve damage.

Women need 2.4 micrograms of vitamin B_{12} daily. Natural B_{12} is found only in animal foods, but after age 50, most of your vitamin B_{12} should be in the synthetic form—the kind that is added to dietary supplements and fortified foods such as breakfast cereals and nutritional yeast. That's because aging decreases levels of stomach acid necessary to absorb the natural form of vitamin B_{12}, and synthetic vitamin B_{12} doesn't require stomach acid for absorption.

People with celiac or Crohn's disease, and those who have had weight-loss surgery, may absorb less vitamin B_{12}. Common medications like proton pump inhibitors such as Prevacid and Prilosec (omeprazole) can cause vitamin B_{12} deficiency.[33] Ask your doctor or nurse practitioner about the medication you take. You may need extra vitamin B_{12}.

Lutein and Zeaxanthin. Lutein and zeaxanthin are carotenoids, which are natural pigments in food that provide fruits and vegetables, such as corn, spinach, kale, and broccoli, and egg yolks, with their color. Lutein and zeaxanthin accumulate in the retina, where they help protect eyesight by absorbing damaging blue light, reducing inflammation, and deflecting damage from free radicals, which are destructive forms of oxygen in the body. Lutein and zeaxanthin are also present in the brain, including in the hippocampus. Increasingly, lutein and zeaxanthin are garnering attention for their role in cognitive function, although the relationship is stronger for lutein, as it is the predominant carotenoid in our brain.[34]

Eating at least six servings a week of leafy greens and including eggs on a regular basis provide significant amounts of lutein and zeaxanthin, which is easy to do on the Menopause Diet Plan.

More Ways to Save Your Brain

It may take years or decades to develop Alzheimer's disease and other dementias, making it difficult to determine exactly which habits affect the course of these conditions. Most of the associations between lifestyle and brain health come from observations of large groups of people, not clinical trials. Even so, it's helpful to make the healthiest choices possible to safeguard your brain. Here are some suggestions:

Achieve and maintain a healthy weight. Body fat churns out hormones and compounds that trigger inflammation, and it contributes to high blood pressure, elevated cholesterol levels, and diabetes—all of which harm the brain.

Get enough quality sleep. Sleep is vital to brain health. When you're tired, especially on a daily basis, it's more difficult to form or maintain the pathways that allow you to learn and create memories. It's also harder to concentrate and process information as quickly as when you're well rested. Emerging evidence from animal studies suggests that sleep is necessary to clear toxins associated with the build-up of plaques seen with Alzheimer's disease.[35] Sleep apnea is a condition that causes breathing to stop briefly and frequently when asleep. Left untreated, sleep apnea may contribute to memory loss and dementia.[36] If you're having difficulties getting the rest you need, talk with a sleep specialist.

Mind your medications. Review all the medications you take with your doctor or nurse practitioner. Long-term use of a class of medications called anticholinergics has been associated with a higher risk of dementia. One study comparing the medical records of 40,770 people older than 65 diagnosed with dementia and 283,933 seniors without the condition found those with dementia were up to 30% more likely to have been prescribed anticholinergic medications for Parkinson's disease, bladder problems, or depression.[37] Ask your doctor, nurse practitioner, or pharmacist if you are taking anticholinergic medications. Statin drugs, which people take to lower LDL cholesterol levels, may also result in memory problems.[38] We're not advising you to stop taking prescribed medications to protect your brain health. However, it's a good idea to consider both the risks and the benefits of medication, including the over-the-counter kind, and to work on lifestyle changes that limit medication use.

Limit alcohol intake. The Mediterranean eating pattern includes small amounts of wine every day, but the Menopause Diet Plan does not, although wine is not off-limits. While moderate alcohol intake, defined as less than one drink per day for a woman, may help the heart and the brain, heavy alcohol consumption has been associated with changes in brain structures, cognitive impairments, and an increased risk of all types of dementia.[39]

Maintain your social networks. Evidence from the Northwestern University SuperAging Program suggests that cognitive decline doesn't occur in everyone. In one study, those with a strong network of friends and family performed as well or better than people twenty to thirty years younger on tests of episodic memory, the type of memory that declines with aging and drops off dramatically in Alzheimer's dementia.[40]

Be good to your gut. The gut has its own nervous system that it uses to signal the brain, and the two "talk" all day long. Food, medication, and chronic conditions affect communication along the gut-brain axis and may trigger inflammation in brain cells.

6

CURBING CANCER RISK

> There's a history of cancer in my family and getting older was a reminder I should be doing all I can to prevent it.
>
> —*Sally, age 59*

Menopause does not cause cancer. However, cancer risk does increase during and after the menopause transition because women are getting older. Several diet and lifestyle factors that become more common through the peri- and postmenopausal years can also potentially increase cancer risk due to their influence on diet quality, including the following:

- Weight gain, particularly an excess accumulation of belly fat
- A more sedentary lifestyle
- Less meal planning and more dining out (and drinking!) now that the kids are older
- Lack of time due to stresses common in midlife, such as work stress or caring for aging parents, that may trigger a shift away from fruits and vegetables and toward the convenience or comfort of highly processed foods

Cancers can take years, even decades, to develop, and scientific research shows that risk is a combination of our genes, lifestyle, and environment. While we can't change our DNA, we can influence our diet, physical activity, and other lifestyle habits, as well as possibly the environment in which we live and work, although we realize that's not an option available to everyone.

Historically, whether a person developed cancer or not was largely considered a matter of luck—or the lack of it. Now, thanks to the hard work of researchers and organizations around the world committed to studying cancer prevention, we understand there's a lot we can do to lower cancer risk. According to the American Institute for Cancer Research (AICR), an organization whose mission is to fund research and provide education about diet, lifestyle, and cancer prevention, around 40% of cancers are preventable by not smoking and with other healthy habits.[1]

Let's start with a discussion of how cancer develops to enhance your understanding of how a balanced diet and other positive lifestyle habits may lower your risk.

What Is Cancer?

According to the National Cancer Institute (NCI),[2] cancer is a collection of related diseases that have in common a state whereby some of the body's cells begin to divide without stopping, eventually spreading into surrounding tissues.

Our body contains trillions of cells, all of which are constantly growing and dividing to form new cells. Under normal conditions, when cells get old or become damaged, they die off and new cells take their place. This orderly process usually marches on, day in and day out, without incident, unless something goes wrong and skews things. Cancer can develop almost anywhere in the body where either cells that are abnormal or damaged don't die off or new cells form where they shouldn't. For reasons we don't fully understand, these abnormal or excess cells can divide without stopping, ultimately taking shape as growths called *tumors*.

Many cancers form solid tumors, although cancers of the blood, like leukemia, generally do not. Cancerous tumors are malignant, which means they can invade nearby tissues. As these tumors grow, some cancer cells can break off and travel to distant places in the body through the blood or lymph system and form new tumors far from the original site. These are called *metastases*.

Although we often talk about cancer as if it's one condition affecting different body parts, there are actually over 100 types, some of which appear to be influenced by lifestyle, some not. Of those without a clear connection to diet and lifestyle, it could be they affect fewer people so researchers haven't studied them as much as more common cancers.

How Do Types of Cancer Differ?

Most of the more common cancers are solid-tumor cancers and are usually named for the organs or tissues where they form, like lung, brain, or colon cancer. Cancers may also be described by their cell type, such as epithelial or squamous cell cancer.

Cancers are mostly broken down into these major types. While these are the most frequently diagnosed cancers, many other forms exist:

- Carcinomas are the most common type of cancer. They are formed by cells that cover the inside and outside surfaces of the body. These include adenocarcinomas (most breast, prostate, pancreatic, colon cancers); basal cell carcinomas (skin cancer); and squamous cell carcinoma (including skin, throat, stomach, intestines, lungs, bladder, and kidneys).

- Sarcomas form in bone and soft tissues, including muscle, fat, and blood vessels.
- Leukemia begins in the bones. Abnormal white blood cells build up in the blood and bone marrow, crowding out normal blood cells.
- Lymphoma starts in the lymphocytes, which are disease-fighting white blood cells that are part of the immune system.
- Melanoma originates in cells that give skin its color.
- Brain and spinal cord tumors are named based on the type of cells they contain and where in the central nervous system they develop.

What Are the Differences Between Cancer Cells and Normal Cells?

Cancer cells differ from normal cells in many ways that allow them to grow out of control and become invasive. Cancer cells are less specialized than normal cells. Whereas normal cells mature into very specific cell types with specific functions, cancer cells don't. This is one reason cancer cells continue to divide without stopping.

For reasons we don't fully understand, cancer cells are able to evade signals that normally tell cells to stop dividing and begin a process known as "programmed cell death," which the body uses to destroy abnormal cells. Cancer cells also have a unique ability to stimulate nearby normal cells to form small blood vessels, called capillaries, that can supply tumors with the oxygen and nutrients they need to grow. This abnormal capillary growth is called *angiogenesis* and is the target of a category of chemotherapy drugs, the idea being to block abnormal cells from accessing nutrients and other elements for growth.

Cancer cells are also often able to evade the immune system, a network of specialized cells that protect the body from infections and other health problems. Although the immune system normally targets damaged or abnormal cells for destruction, some cancer cells can sneak by, enabling them to continue to grow. Tumors can also use the immune system to stay alive and reproduce with the help of certain immune system cells that are designed to prevent a runaway immune response (which can cause autoimmune conditions like rheumatoid arthritis). Cancerous cells can exploit this process, protecting themselves from destruction by the immune system.

What Causes Cancer to Develop?

Cancer is a genetic disease—that is, it is caused by changes to genes that control the way our cells function, especially how they grow and divide. Genetic changes that cause cancer can be inherited (such as the BRCA genes associated with breast and ovarian cancer) and can arise over a lifetime of errors that occur as cells divide, or from damage to our genes caused by exposure to smoking, radiation (at work or during cancer treatment), and ultraviolet light from the sun. In general, cancer cells have more genetic changes than normal cells, and each person's cancer has a unique combination of genetic alterations. Scientists are busy trying to understand these genetic influences, as they also make good targets for cancer-fighting drugs.

Damaged cells that turn into cancer can emerge from a number of ongoing internal processes, including oxidation. Oxidation is a natural process that can fight infection, but too much oxidation is harmful. Ideally, excess oxidation is neutralized by *anti*oxidant compounds, including certain vitamins, such as vitamins C and E, minerals such as selenium, and phytonutrients, or beneficial substances found in fruits, vegetables, whole grains, nuts, seeds, legumes, herbs, and spices like turmeric. Unfortunately, modern life is loaded with oxidizing influences, such as smoking, exposure to secondhand smoke, and air pollution, and most of us have diets that are sorely lacking in plant foods. When there is an imbalance between oxidation and antioxidant activity, cells become vulnerable not only to cancer but also to other conditions like diabetes and cardiovascular and neurologic diseases.

Similar to oxidation, inflammation is an important force designed to promote healing by shuttling nutrients and immune cells to the site of an infection or injury, but when left unchecked, inflammation is tied to most modern-day health problems. Plant-based diets and seafood provide anti-inflammatory nutrients to control inflammation. Unfortunately, modern life triggers inflammation that often settles in, potentially causing cell damage that can lead to cancer and other pro-inflammatory health problems.[3] Extra fat in the belly and other places makes matters worse by creating a pro-inflammatory, pro-oxidative environment in the body.

Why Diet and Lifestyle Choices Matter for Cancer Prevention

Diet, weight status, and lifestyle choices such as regular exercise, smoking, and drinking alcohol to excess can influence cancer risk by either positively or negatively affecting the environment in the body where cells are growing and dividing. Our immune system is tasked with defending us against negative influences, but without enough "backup" from heathy diet and lifestyle factors, it can become overwhelmed by too many challenges.

It's important to understand how cancer cells grow because we *all* have abnormal cells in our body. Fortunately, those abnormal cells usually die before developing into cancer because of the body's strong defense system. Our immune system, aided by antioxidant and anti-inflammatory nutrients, tries to contend with abnormal cells by neutralizing oxidation, quelling inflammation, and assisting our liver and kidneys with detoxification of potentially harmful substances. Healthful habits, such as eating more plant foods and seafood, cutting back on added sugars and highly processed choices, and engaging in some daily exercise, contribute to cancer defense by "walling off" abnormal cells so they're unable to grow and develop. The "bricks" in that wall are antioxidants, anti-inflammatory nutrients, immune cells, and other elements involved in keeping cell replication normal. We can't change our genetics, but we can take steps to boost our natural defense against cancer.

Besides lowering cancer risk, making positive changes in your diet, lifestyle, and body weight lowers the risk of all kinds of diseases associated with inflammation, oxidation, and other harmful influences, like smoking. Lifestyle habits for reducing your cancer risk are the same before, during, and after menopause. Let's look closely at how each of these factors may make you more, or less, vulnerable to cancer.

What Works for Us

I can't stress enough how critical it is to understand there are many people who eat healthy, exercise regularly, and maintain a healthy weight and still get cancer. This speaks to the complexity of this disease and influences we don't fully understand. But, as with disease prevention in general, ample evidence exists that many cancers are preventable, so developing cancer-fighting diet and lifestyle habits are an important part of hedging your bets.

—Hillary

AICR GENERAL RECOMMENDATIONS TO REDUCE CANCER RISK

Three times over the last twenty years, the AICR, in partnership with the World Cancer Research Fund (WCRF), has updated their cancer prevention recommendations based on a massive international analysis of the latest available research on diet, nutrition, physical activity, and cancer. Owing to escalating interest in cancer prevention, with each review there have been thousands more studies to consider. Since 2007, the review has also included an exploding amount of research on cancer survivorship.

The AICR/WCRF rely on only high-quality data to inform their recommendations, which are considered the gold standard for the science on cancer prevention. Scientists gather all the in-depth research on diet, physical activity, and lifestyle topics related to cancer and farm them out to experts on different kinds of cancers for feedback. All recommendations must be backed by a solid amount of supportive evidence, with a goal of clarifying for laypeople what cancer-prevention information appears "real." This mission of the AICR/WCRF is critical, as much of what people read about diet and cancer on the Internet is hearsay more than science, and that hearsay often generates more fear than hope about preventing cancer.

The 2018 Ten Cancer Prevention Recommendations for general cancer prevention are available online at the AICR website, https://www.aicr.org/reduce-your-cancer-risk/recommendations -for-cancer-prevention/index.html. We summarize them here and offer some explanation:

1. Be at a healthy weight: Keep your weight within a healthy range and avoid weight gain in adult life.

According to the AICR, next to not smoking, maintaining a healthy weight is the most important thing you can do to reduce your cancer risk, as overwhelming evidence has linked excess body fat with an overall increased risk of cancer.[4]

Excess weight is clearly linked with cancers of the breast (in postmenopausal women only), colon, rectum, endometrium, esophagus, kidney, and pancreas. Being overweight might also raise the risk of cancers of the gallbladder, liver, and cervix, as well as aggressive prostate cancer. In addition, excess belly fat, regardless of total body weight, is linked with an increased risk of colorectal cancer and may play a role in cancers of the pancreas, endometrium, and breast (in women past menopause).[5]

Why excess weight is linked with increased breast cancer risk in postmenopausal women, but not in the premenopausal years, isn't clear. However, body fat affects physiology. We've long thought of excess body fat as just stored calories, but now we know that fat doesn't just sit there on our waists, butt, and thighs. Fat is a metabolic organ that can encourage the growth of abnormal cells and wreak havoc on health, for the following reasons:

- Excess body fat can trigger insulin resistance (see chapter 4 for more on this topic), which in turn increases circulating levels of insulin and other hormones that encourage the growth of abnormal cells.
- Body fat produces estrogen, which may contribute to the growth of breast and other hormone-sensitive cancers.
- Excess body fat promotes inflammation and oxidation, which, when not neutralized, can damage cells, leaving them vulnerable to cancerous changes.
- Obesity may contribute to a state where it's possible for abnormal cells to evade our body's usual mechanisms for promoting cell deaths and alter the immune response that normally contributes to this process.

Can weight loss later in life turn this ship around? Research on whether losing weight lowers cancer risk is limited, but increasing evidence suggests that weight loss might reduce the risk of postmenopausal breast cancer, more aggressive forms of prostate cancer, and possibly other cancers, too. In fact, strong evidence backs up the value of maintaining a healthy weight in avoiding breast cancer. One review of 139 studies on the role of physical activity and weight loss on breast cancer risk found that losing weight was associated with a lower incidence of the disease. Physical activity was tied to a significantly lower risk of breast cancer in both pre- and postmenopausal women, with high intensity exercise being slightly more protective.[6]

Of course, the ideal situation is to strive to maintain the healthiest weight you can throughout life. But given that overweight people who intentionally lose weight have reduced levels of the hormones related to cancer risk, such as insulin and estrogen, and weight loss reduces inflammation, it follows that body changes that occur with weight loss may, indeed, reduce cancer risk.

2. Be physically active as part of everyday life—walk more, sit less.

Research has demonstrated that physical activity lowers the risk of breast, colon, endometrial, liver, and esophageal cancer, and may improve survivorship after a breast cancer diagnosis. Given its role in promoting a healthy weight, we think it's safe to say that being physically active is very effective for preventing cancer and for survivorship. Physical activity helps lower cancer risk in several ways:

- It keeps hormone levels, including insulin and other growth hormones that in excess may encourage cancer growth, in a healthy range.
- It strengthens the immune system.
- It speeds the movement of food through the intestinal tract, limiting the gut's exposure to potentially harmful substances in food.
- It may help to avoid weight gain, which increases the risk of many cancer types.

The AICR, the NCI, and the American Cancer Society (ACS) all recommend at least 150 minutes of moderate physical activity, or 75 minutes of vigorous activity, or equivalent combination of both, preferably spread throughout the week. For cancer prevention and weight control, higher levels of activity provide even more benefit. Work toward achieving 45 to 60 minutes of moderate-intensity physical activity daily. Going beyond 60 minutes daily provides additional health benefits.

Although physical activity recommendations for cancer prevention emphasize increasing activity, just sitting less plays an important role. More time spent sitting is linked to weight gain, as well as to higher levels of belly fat, insulin, and blood sugar, exposing the body's cells to more growth hormones, day in and day out. But, also, any physical activity is better than none. Even 10 minutes of walking bestows some health benefits, but if you can do more exercise, you should.

Everything you want to know about physical activity and health—and how to incorporate a doable plan into your life—is covered in detail in chapter 9.

3. Eat a diet rich in whole grains, fruits, vegetables and beans: Make whole grains, vegetables, fruits, and pulses (legumes), such as beans and lentils, a major part of your usual diet.

Research continuously points to clear connections between what we eat and our risk of getting cancer. When preparing a meal, aim to fill at least two-thirds of your plate with vegetables, fruits, whole grains, and beans. In addition to vitamins and minerals, plant foods are good sources of phytonutrients.

In our "super foods" world, we like to think specific foods either cause cancer ("artificial sweeteners!") or fight it ("eat blueberries!"). In reality, the science linking artificial sweeteners to cancer is lacking (though there are other reasons to limit their use, as discussed in chapter 4).[7] Also, it's impossible to discern the role of specific foods in cancer prevention, as we consume thousands of dietary components each day, with the typical diet providing more than 25,000 physiologically active food elements.[8]

Certain vitamins and minerals, and healthy fats, play a role in cancer prevention. But most cancer-fighting food compounds belong to a category of over 100,000 nutrients found in plants called phytonutrients (*phyto* means "plant" in Greek), which are naturally occurring elements in fruits, vegetables, whole grains, nuts, seeds, legumes, tea leaves, coffee beans, herbs, and spices. Phytonutrients give plants their color (hence the benefits of eating blueberries) and act as the plant's immune system, performing antioxidant, anti-inflammatory, and detoxifying duties. When we eat plants, we also benefit from their phytonutrients, which enhance our immune system's ability to defend us. Phytonutrients (and dietary fiber) are likely responsible for most of the health benefits tied to eating a more plant-based diet.

In summary, food supplies an array of compounds with the potential to intervene in multiple aspects of the cancer process, alone or in combination with other nutrients, making it impossible to assign specific health effects to individual foods. This effect supports what we know to be true about nutrition in general—overall dietary patterns matter most, not the occasional consumption of any single food, which is the "80/20" rule in action!

Is Soy Okay to Eat?

Soy is a healthy plant-based protein that has been widely studied for its association with cancer. Animal studies once suggested that isoflavones, a weak plant form of estrogen found in soy, might be harmful for breast cancer survivors. Fortunately, large human studies now support a consistent body of research showing that soy foods are safe to consume, even with a cancer diagnosis. Studies looking at soy intake and breast cancer survivorship have concluded that consuming moderate amounts of soy is not associated with a higher risk of recurrence or of death. This advice applies to whole-food forms of soy—tofu, tempeh, miso, edamame, and soy milk—not pills, powders, or bars, which, as concentrated forms of soy, may behave differently than whole soy foods.

4. Limit consumption of fast foods and other processed foods high in fat, starches, and sugars. Eating less of these foods helps control calorie intake and maintain a healthy weight.

There is strong evidence that consuming fast foods and a Western-type diet contribute to overweight and obesity, which is linked to twelve types of cancer. Eating fewer highly processed foods creates more room in your diet for fiber-rich, plant-based choices.

Why Fiber Helps Reduce Cancer Risk

According to the AICR, foods containing dietary fiber, such as vegetables, fruits, legumes, and whole grains, may protect against cancers of the mouth, pharynx, larynx, esophagus, colon, rectum, and stomach. Fiber helps to manage blood glucose and insulin levels, aids in weight control, speeds the passage of harmful substances through the intestines, and produces substances that protect the lining of the colon. Dietary fiber also nurtures a healthy gut microbiome, which science suggests plays a role in maintaining a cancer-fighting immune response.[9] For cancer prevention, AICR recommends aiming for about 30 grams of dietary fiber daily, or about double what the average American consumes.[10] To reach that goal, try to include at least five servings of fruits and vegetables and three servings of whole grains. You might be surprised by the many benefits you feel after boosting your fiber intake!

5. Limit consumption of red and processed meat. Eat only moderate amounts of red meat, such as beef, pork, and lamb. Eat little, if any, processed meat.

The evidence that red meat is a cause of colorectal cancer is convincing, but studies show we can consume modest amounts—12 to 18 ounces (cooked) per week—without a measurable increase in risk. For processed meat (ham, bacon, salami, hot dogs, sausages), convincing evidence suggests that cancer risk begins to increase with even very low consumption.

6. Limit consumption of sugar-sweetened drinks. Opt for mostly water and unsweetened drinks.

There is strong evidence that consuming sugar-sweetened beverages causes weight gain, which is linked to twelve types of cancer.

7. Limit alcohol consumption. For cancer prevention, it's best not to drink alcohol.

Alcohol in any form is a carcinogen, or cancer-causing agent. Alcohol is linked to cancers of mouth, pharynx, larynx, esophagus, liver, breast, stomach, and colorectum.[11] The best advice for those concerned about cancer is not to drink, but if you choose to do so, limit your consumption to one drink per day for women and two for men. See chapter 8 for more on drink serving sizes.

8. Do not use supplements for cancer prevention. Aim to meet nutritional needs through diet alone.

The AICR doesn't discourage the use of specific supplements for those who may benefit, such as pregnant women and the elderly, but they caution against expecting any dietary supplement to lower cancer risk as well as a healthy diet. Also, high-dose beta-carotene supplements have been linked to an increased risk of lung cancer in current and former smokers, so we can't assume that high-dose supplementation of any kind is safe. See more about dietary supplements in chapter 10.

Dietary Supplements and Cancer

Studies show the majority of Americans have used dietary supplements at one time or another. While some situations may call for supplements to fill nutrient voids in the diet—as in pregnancy or a vitamin or mineral deficiency—evidence is lacking that taking dietary supplements either lowers the risk of getting cancer or improves survivorship. Some research suggests that high-dose antioxidant supplementation may compete with cancer treatment (although these findings are considered inconclusive) or protect abnormal cells from targeted destruction, as was assumed to be the case with studies showing beta-carotene supplement users who smoked had higher rates of lung cancer.[12] After treatment, a woman may need supplementation to treat deficiencies that arise during treatment, but research shows supplements do not offer cancer protection or benefits for survivors. Although taking a basic multivitamin/mineral supplement is unlikely to be harmful, at this point there just isn't enough research to weigh the benefits of high-dose supplementation against potential harms.[13] An exception may be vitamin D. One recent large study suggested higher blood levels of vitamin D were associated with significantly lower risk of colorectal cancer in women.[14] This doesn't provide support for universal vitamin D supplementation to prevent cancer but does suggest it's important not to be deficient. As vitamin D is involved with keeping cell replication normal, for those with a cancer diagnosis it's reasonable to request a blood test to check for a deficiency.[15]

9. For mothers, breastfeed your baby if you can. Breastfeeding is good for both mother and baby.

We know you're beyond your breastfeeding days, but this is good information to pass along. There is strong evidence that breast-feeding helps protect against breast cancer in the mother, likely for two reasons: First, breastfeeding lowers the levels of some cancer-related hormones in mom, and, second, it gets rid of cells in the breast that may have damaged DNA. In addition, babies who are breastfed are less likely to become overweight.

10. After a cancer diagnosis, follow recommendations for cancer prevention as much as possible.

Once treatment has been completed, evidence suggests the same strategies that may reduce your risk of getting cancer also appear beneficial for cancer survivorship. Maintain the healthiest weight you can, opt for a more plant-based diet low in red and processed meat and added sugar, and prioritize physical activity on as many days as possible during the week.

For those who want more details, the entire report informing the recommendations can be found at the AICR website, www.aicr.org.

What Works for Us

As a nutritionist who's worked with patients during and after cancer treatment for over thirty years, it's clear to me that eating as healthfully as possible, hydrating well, and maintaining physical activity may improve not only survivorship but also quality of life, both physically and mentally. Even if a woman's cancer isn't curable, tending to the rest of her body aside from the treatment may help her enjoy each day a little more.

—Hillary

Recommendations by Cancer Type for Menopausal Women

Research from the AICR suggests that the cancers more strongly influenced by diet and lifestyle in women are breast, colorectal, endometrial, and ovarian cancers.

BREAST CANCER

Aside from skin cancer, breast cancer is the most common cancer in women, and the older a woman is, the more likely she is to get breast cancer. Thanks to advocacy, breast cancer has been studied extensively for diet and lifestyle influences. The AICR has identified the following as factors that affect breast cancer risk:[16]

- Alcohol increases levels of estrogen and other hormones that make cancer more likely.
- Excess body fat causes inflammation and increases blood levels of insulin and other growth hormones that boost cancer risk.
- Physical activity decreases breast cancer risk by helping with weight management and regulating insulin and other hormone levels. Being physically active before and after diagnosis may increase cancer survival.
- Plant-based diets help with weight management and provide numerous cancer-fighting nutrients.
- Having breastfed reduces breast cancer risk by helping the body to get rid of cells with damaged DNA. Don't be concerned if you didn't breastfeed, however. For breast cancer prevention, the other facts listed here carry much more weight.

COLORECTAL CANCER

The risk of colorectal cancer (CRC) increases with age. According to the AICR, excess body fat, consuming processed meats and high amounts of red meat, and drinking two or more alcohol-containing drinks per day raise the risk for CRC. Eating whole grains, fruits, vegetables, legumes, nuts and seeds, garlic, and other foods containing fiber, as well as daily moderate physical activity, lowers the risk.[17]

ENDOMETRIAL CANCER

Endometrial cancer is the most common cancer of the female reproductive tract, accounting for more cases of cancer each year than ovarian and cervical cancers combined. Most cases are diagnosed in women over age 60. Being overweight, being sedentary, having type 2 diabetes, or receiving a diagnosis of polycystic ovary syndrome are considered risk factors.[18]

Eating a diet high in refined carbohydrates and sugary drinks also increases endometrial cancer risk by aggravating insulin resistance. Factors associated with a lower risk of endometrial cancer include physical activity, drinking coffee (yay!), and maintaining a healthy weight.[19]

OVARIAN CANCER

Ovarian cancer is the seventh most common cancer in women worldwide, with higher rates in high-income countries like the United States. Risk increases with age, although the rate of increase actually slows after menopause. According to the AICR, having higher levels of body fat is a probable cause of ovarian cancer, making it one more cancer that may be influenced by maintaining a healthy weight.[20]

Does Sugar Feed Cancer?

Anyone with a cancer diagnosis has undoubtedly been cautioned to avoid sugar because "sugar feeds cancer." There are many reasons to limit added sugar, including its connection to weight gain, a risk factor for several cancers. But saying that sugar feeds cancer is an oversimplification of a complex issue. Like excess intake of any carbohydrate, regularly consuming too much added sugar will result in greater fluctuations in blood glucose levels, which stimulates greater insulin secretion. Insulin is a growth hormone that makes cells grow whether or not they are cancerous. The key is the quantity—smaller amounts of sweets eaten occasionally as treats will cause temporary blips in your blood sugar and insulin, whereas regular intake of large amounts of sugar will more consistently expose your body's cells to elevations of insulin.

7

BETTER YOUR
BONE HEALTH

My mother had osteoporosis, and it took a toll on her
quality of life. Hopefully, I can avoid what she went
through because we know so much more about it now.
—Annemarie, age 49

There's more to your bones than meets the eye. From the outside, bones appear strong and rigid, and it seems they do
little more than provide structure for the body and protect
vital organs. But on the inside, bones are teeming with activity.
Their tough exteriors harbor tissue that is constantly churning out
cells that carry oxygen, fight infection, and aid in blood clotting.
Bones also serve as a storehouse for minerals that provide skeletal
strength and support health.

As you may have guessed, menopause presents a challenge to
bone health. The good news is that it's never too late to take better
care of your bones.

All About Bones

In the years before and during puberty, your bones got longer as
you grew taller. They became thicker, too, while continuing to accumulate mass long after you reached your adult height. At around

age 30, your skeleton achieved maximum strength and density, known as peak bone mass, and until that time, your body made new bone cells at a relatively rapid pace.[1] After 30, you gradually started to lose bone mass. Declining levels of estrogen during perimenopause and menopause, as well as ovary removal, result in the formation of fewer new bone cells, which ultimately weakens bones. Women lose the most bone tissue in the first few years after menopause. After that, bone loss continues at a slower pace for the rest of their lives.

We know the situation sounds grim. Everyone loses bone with age, but it's the amount that counts. It's best to have as much bone tissue as possible before menopause starts. Very low bone mass is a risk for osteoporosis, often referred to as brittle bone disease.[2]

What Is Osteoporosis?

We all know at least one older woman who has become shorter with age. Maybe your mom, an elderly aunt, or a neighbor has fallen and fractured a hip. Chances are, osteoporosis is to blame. Of the estimated 10 million Americans with osteoporosis, about 80% of them are women.[3]

Osteoporosis is a chronic condition marked by very low bone density that sets the stage for bone fracture, particularly in the hip, spine, wrist, and forearm. The inside of osteoporotic bones features large gaps in bone tissue. In osteoporosis, most broken bones are caused by falls, but the condition can weaken the skeleton so much that it's possible to fracture a bone simply by coughing or bumping into a piece of furniture. Osteoporosis is also linked to loose teeth and tooth loss.[4]

Experts estimate that, in addition to those with osteoporosis, an additional 43 million adults, also mostly women, have low bone density. Low bone density is when bone density measures below normal levels, but not low enough to be classified as osteoporosis.[5] Low bone density increases the risk for bone fracture. Breaking a bone for any reason before age 50 should be taken seriously because it may signal low bone mass.[6]

Risk Factors for Osteoporosis

Osteoporosis is often referred to as a silent disease because there are typically no symptoms of bone loss. You may not know you have osteoporosis until your bones become weak enough to break.

While menopause accelerates bone loss, it doesn't mean osteoporosis is in your future. Many factors contribute to bone health, and some of them are under your control while others are not. For example, you can't change the fact that you're a woman experiencing perimenopause or menopause, you're a Caucasian or Asian woman, or you have a small body frame, all of which increase the risk for osteoporosis.[7]

You also can't do much about your health history, but it pays to be aware that certain conditions are linked to weaker bones, including diabetes, inflammatory bowel disease, liver disease, kidney disease, multiple sclerosis, and rheumatoid arthritis.

How to Boost Bone Strength

Years of inadequate calcium and vitamin D intake, and a sedentary lifestyle, can interfere with achieving and maintaining maximal bone mass. But that's water under the bridge. Concentrate on what you can control about bone health from now on, including eating a balanced diet that has enough of these bone-building nutrients.

CALCIUM

Calcium is the most abundant mineral in the body. Calcium helps maintain heart rhythm, muscle contraction, and efficient communication among nerve cells. It's the major structural component of bones, and the bones serve as a calcium reserve.

The body relies on the calcium in bones to maintain the correct calcium levels in the muscle, blood, and other bodily fluids. When calcium intake is low, or when your body doesn't absorb enough calcium, or both, the body withdraws the calcium it needs from the bones. A steady, adequate intake of calcium allows the body to repay the bones to maintain calcium reserves. Menopause hastens calcium loss from the bones, forcing the body to make more withdrawals of calcium from the skeleton than deposits, which chips away at bone strength.[8]

Consuming adequate calcium helps maintain bone mass. After age 50, the body absorbs less calcium from food and dietary supplements. To account for the decline, the suggested daily intake for calcium increases by 200 milligrams (mg) daily to 1,200 milligrams per day, which can come from food, dietary supplements, or a combination.[9]

Dairy foods are naturally rich in calcium, and fortified beverages, including orange juice and soy milk, may also provide bone-building calcium and vitamin D. Dark green leafy vegetables, such as Chinese cabbage, kale, and broccoli, contain calcium, but the body doesn't absorb it as well as the calcium in dairy foods and certain supplements. If you don't get enough calcium from foods on a daily basis, you may need a dietary supplement to fill in gaps that could help prevent broken bones. See chapter 10 for more on calcium supplements.

FOOD TYPE	AMOUNT OF CALCIUM (MG)
Tofu, firm, prepared with calcium (¼ block)	553
Yogurt, plain, fat-free (1 cup)	452
Soy milk, fortified (Silk brand Original)	450
Orange juice, calcium added (8 ounces)	364
Yogurt, fruit-flavored, low-fat (1 cup)	345
Milk, plain (1 cup)	305
Yogurt, Greek, plain, low-fat (1 cup)	262
Cheddar cheese (1 ounce)	201
Cottage cheese, 1% low-fat (½ cup)	99
Broccoli, chopped (1 cup), cooked	62

Source: U.S. Department of Agriculture, Agricultural Research Service, U.S.D.A. Food Composition Databases; available at https://ndb.nal.usda.gov/ndb/.

What Works for Us

I have a confession. While I love dairy foods, I don't typically consume four servings daily, the amount that helps provide the calcium I need as a woman over 50. At the end of the day, I figure out what I need to take as a supplement to make up for what I missed in food, and it's typically one 600-milligram calcium pill.

—Liz

VITAMIN D

Consuming adequate amounts of vitamin D is just as important as getting enough calcium to support bone health. That's because vitamin D maximizes the body's absorption of calcium from food and dietary supplements and regulates calcium's movement in and out of bones to maintain calcium balance in the body.

Unlike calcium, the body makes vitamin D. Production begins when skin is exposed to strong ultraviolet B (UVB) rays from the sun, and it ends in the liver and kidneys. It's possible to produce and store all the vitamin D necessary for a year with a few minutes of direct exposure to the sun a few times a week during the summer months.[10]

Though vitamin D production in the body contributes to meeting needs, most people do not make enough vitamin D. In addition, many women fail to get what they need from food. There are several reasons why vitamin D levels may be low in your body, including the following:

- Using sunscreen with an SPF of 8 and above, which blocks most or all of the UVB rays necessary for vitamin D production.
- Having darker skin, which contains melanin, a compound that decreases the production of vitamin D in response to UVB rays.
- Being overweight. Research suggests that people with a BMI of ≥ 30 may need more vitamin D than those with a lower BMI for optimal blood levels.
- Aging. The body is less efficient at making vitamin D as you get older.
- Limiting vitamin D-rich foods. People with milk allergy, lactose intolerance, or who follow a vegan diet or other eating plans that limit certain foods may have insufficient vitamin D intake.

Salmon and tuna are excellent sources of natural vitamin D. Dairy milk and plant milks including soy, oat, and almond are often fortified with vitamin D. Eggs from hens who eat vitamin D-rich feed supply the nutrient, too. Most brands of yogurt and cheese do not contain added vitamin D, however, so check the label.

Suggested vitamin D intakes and levels in food are expressed in both micrograms (mcg) and International Units (IUs). Everyone from ages 1 to 71 needs 15 mcg (600 IU) of vitamin D daily, and 20 mcg (800 IU) daily after age 71.[11] If it's not possible to get enough vitamin D from food and sunshine, consider dietary supplements to fill in gaps. If you develop a vitamin D deficiency, you'll initially need a higher dose of vitamin D to restore your levels to normal. After that, it's important to get adequate amounts of vitamin D regularly to avoid becoming deficient again. Tell your doctor or nurse practitioner if you are taking vitamin D supplements, as they can interact with several common medications, including prednisone and cholestyramine.

FOOD TYPE	AMOUNT OF VITAMIN D MCG/IU
Salmon (sockeye), cooked (3 ounces)	14/570
Tuna, light, canned, drained (3 ounces)	5/216
Soy beverage, fortified, all flavors, unsweetened (8 ounces)	3/119
Orange juice, vitamin D–fortified (8 ounces)	2.5/100
Egg (1), fortified	2.5/100
Milk, fortified, 1% low-fat (8 ounces)	2.5/100
Yogurt, fortified (5 ounces)	2/74
Egg (1), large	1/41

Source: U.S. Department of Agriculture, Agricultural Research Service, U.S.D.A. Food Composition Databases; available at https://ndb.nal .usda.gov/ndb/.

MAGNESIUM

Bone is the home to about half of all the magnesium in the body, and the rest is divided among other tissues and organs. Only 1% of the magnesium is in the blood, but that level is critical, as magnesium contributes to about 300 bodily functions.[12] Magnesium is found in greater amounts in plant foods, such as legumes, nuts, seeds, vegetables, and whole grains. Foods rich in magnesium also contain potassium and fiber, two nutrients that play a role in overall wellness.

The suggested daily magnesium intake for women over the age of 31 is 320 milligrams. Surveys suggest that many Americans don't get the recommended amounts of magnesium. Magnesium deficiency is linked to lower bone density.[13]

While it's preferable to get nutrients from food, the amount of magnesium in a regular multivitamin/mineral supplement can be helpful for bridging small gaps in your diet. Many popular over-the-counter antacids and laxatives contain magnesium and, when taken frequently, may provide excess magnesium. Consult your doctor or nurse practitioner if you find yourself taking these medications often.[14] Here's how to get the magnesium you need from food.

FOOD TYPE	AMOUNT OF MAGNESIUM (MG)
Black beans (½ cup), cooked	166
Spinach (1 cup), cooked	157
Pumpkin seeds, roasted (1 ounce)	156
Almonds (1 ounce)	76
Cashews (1 ounce)	74
Soybeans (1 cup), cooked	74
Oatmeal, cooked (½ cup)	65

Quinoa, cooked (½ cup)	59
Artichoke hearts (1 cup), cooked	52
Peanut butter (2 tablespoons)	49
Peanuts (1 ounce)	48
Shredded wheat cereal (1 cup)	48
Baked potato, medium, flesh and skin	48
Yogurt, plain, fat-free (8 ounces)	43

Source: U.S. Department of Agriculture, Agricultural Research Service, U.S.D.A. Food Composition Databases; available at https://ndb.nal .usda.gov/ndb/.

VITAMIN K

Like vitamin D, vitamin K is produced in the body. Beneficial bacteria in your digestive tract churn out vitamin K, which is essential for normal blood clotting and bone health, and is necessary to make one of the main components of bone.

The suggested intake for women over the age of 19 is 90 micrograms (mcg) of vitamin K daily.[15] However, some research suggests higher intakes may be associated with better bone health in older women.[16] In one study, Harvard researchers found that women who consumed at least 110 mcg of vitamin K a day were less likely to break a hip than women who consumed less.[17]

People with celiac disease or ulcerative colitis may have lower vitamin K levels. Certain medications, including anticoagulants, antibiotics, antiseizure drugs, and cholestyramine, interfere with vitamin K. Check with your doctor or nurse practitioner about the effects of the medications you take on vitamin K balance.[18]

Plant foods have the most vitamin K. Include one or more servings per day of broccoli, Brussels sprouts, dark green lettuce, collard greens, or kale to meet the daily suggested intake of vitamin K for women.

FOOD TYPE	AMOUNT OF VITAMIN K (MCG)
Kale (½ cup), cooked	531
Spinach (1 cup), cooked	445
Spinach (1 cup), raw	145
Broccoli (½ cup), cooked	110
Brussels sprouts (½ cup), cooked	109
Asparagus (8 spears), cooked	60
Lettuce, romaine, chopped (1 cup)	48
Peas (1 cup), cooked	41
Blueberries (1 cup)	29
Kiwi (1 medium)	28

Source: U.S. Department of Agriculture, Agricultural Research Service, U.S.D.A. Food Composition Databases; available at https://ndb.nal .usda.gov/ndb/.

VITAMIN C

Your body needs vitamin C for many reasons, including bone health. Vitamin C is involved in the formation of collagen, which is a major part of bone tissue. Studies link higher vitamin C intake with a reduced risk for osteoporosis.[19]

Vitamin C is found naturally in plant foods only. The body can't make or store vitamin C, so it must be consumed on a daily basis. Women require 75 milligrams a day of vitamin C. Smokers need an additional 35 milligrams of vitamin C daily.[20]

Antibiotics, NSAIDs (non-steroidal anti-inflammatory drugs, such as aspirin), and other medications can lower vitamin C levels. Vitamin C may also interact with blood thinners.[21] Tell your doctor or nurse practitioner if you take vitamin C supplements.

FOOD TYPE	AMOUNT OF VITAMIN C (MG)
Red bell pepper, raw, chopped (1 cup)	190
Orange juice (8 ounces)	124
Broccoli, chopped (1 cup), cooked	101
Orange (1 large)	98
Strawberries, sliced (1 cup)	90
Grapefruit sections (1 cup)	72
Kiwi (1)	64
Mango, chopped (1 cup)	60
Cantaloupe, chopped (1 cup)	59

FOOD TYPE	AMOUNT OF VITAMIN C (MG)
Raspberries (1 cup)	32
Tomato (1 medium)	17

Source: U.S. Department of Agriculture, Agricultural Research Service, U.S.D.A. Food Composition Databases; available at https://ndb.nal.usda.gov/ndb/.

PROTEIN

The protein in the food you eat provides the body with the amino acids it needs to build protein-rich hormones, enzymes, bone cells, and other compounds that sustain life. You need adequate protein from animal or plant foods, including soy, as part of a balanced diet with enough calcium to support bone health.[22]

Soy foods, such as tofu, soy milk, and edamame, contain compounds called isoflavones that may benefit bone density by stimulating bone formation and decreasing bone cell loss. Soy isoflavones are similar in structure to estrogen in the body, but it's unclear if eating soy instead of animal protein makes a difference to bone health.[23, 24] Read more about protein in chapter 9.

PHYSICAL ACTIVITY

Regular exercise slows the decline in bone mass. According to the 2018 Physical Activity Guidelines for Americans, physically active people, especially women, appear to have a lower risk of hip fracture as compared to inactive individuals. Exercising regularly at any stage of life helps preserve bone mass.

Exercise stresses bones in a good way. Bone-strengthening activities produce a force that signals the skeleton to generate more cells to make itself stronger and denser. Activities that strengthen bones can be aerobic, like brisk walking or running, or anaerobic, such as training with weights, bars, and bands.

Of course, working out is about more than bone strength. Experts suggest a mixture of aerobic, weight-bearing, and bone-strengthening physical activity that is of moderate or vigorous intensity over a week's time.[25] Learn more about how much and what type of activity is best for you in chapter 9.

What Works for Us

Women are pretty good "cardio" exercisers, but many have trouble adopting a strengthening routine. My go-to is a body pump class a couple of times a week. I do much better when there's awesome music playing and someone is telling me what to do.

—Hillary

Bad to the Bone

In addition to adopting bone-building habits, it's important to be aware of what may be harmful to the bones, too.

ALCOHOL

Is alcohol bad for bones? It's not clear.[26] We know that heavy drinking harms bone health, but a review of research conducted with animals and humans found that light to moderate drinking benefits bones. However, it's possible that the people in the studies had many different types of diets and other lifestyle habits that also affect bone health, which makes it difficult to be absolutely certain about alcohol's effects. Research about alcohol and bone health is ongoing. Until we know for sure, it's a good idea to err on the side of caution when it comes to alcohol, which is discussed in chapter 8.

SODIUM

Consuming too much sodium is not good for your blood pressure, and research suggests that sodium has a negative effect on your bones when calcium consumption is too low.[27] However, in one study, postmenopausal women who consumed about 3,000 milligrams of sodium daily and averaged 1,300 to 1,500 milligrams a day of calcium, which is slightly above the suggested intake, did not experience any detrimental effects to their bones. Read more about sodium in food in chapter 3.[28]

SMOKING

Women who smoke tend to have an earlier menopause than nonsmoking women. Furthermore, there is a direct link between smoking cigarettes and osteoporosis. Smoking decreases bone density, although it's unclear whether women who smoke have lower bone density because they smoke or have other risk factors such as poor diet, low physical activity, or both.[29]

CAFFEINE

Caffeine may cause calcium loss in the urine and may also interfere with the body's absorption of calcium from foods and dietary supplements. Some observational studies have linked drinking a lot of coffee to increased risk for bone fracture. However, others have not found the same effect.

Although a large population-based Swedish study that observed older women for about twenty years found that drinking four cups or more of coffee daily was linked to a very small loss in bone density, coffee did not increase the risk for fracture.[30]

The Dietary Guidelines for Americans suggests no more than 400 milligrams of caffeine daily as part of a healthy eating pattern,[31] which is consistent with studies that find this level presents no harm to bone health, particularly when people consume adequate amounts of calcium.[32]

Measuring Bone Density

Your doctor or nurse practitioner may recommend a bone mineral density (BMD) test to assess bone health. BMD tests can identify low bone mass, determine fracture risk, and measure your response to osteoporosis treatment, such as medications. Dual-energy X-ray absorptiometry, or the DXA test, is similar to an X-ray, but with less radiation. This quick, safe, and painless test takes stock of bone density at your hip and spine. Women who are younger than 65 and at high risk for fractures should have a bone density test and so should every woman over age 65.[33] Talk with your healthcare provider about how frequently you should have your bone density measured.

8

THINK YOUR DRINK

During my transition to menopause, I found I needed to drink less alcohol, which I realized was aggravating my night sweats.

—*Marion, age 57*

We humans are nearly all fluid, and every cell in our body requires water to function. Fluid is so important that we've devoted a whole chapter to it. Why? Because in our experience many people aren't aware that fluid affects how they feel. And by people, we mean menopausal women.

Inadequate hydration can worsen fatigue and constipation—common side effects of the transition to menopause. It may also aggravate bloating, which some menopausal women experience. According to the Centers for Disease Control and Prevention (CDC), the likelihood of drinking fewer than 4 cups of water daily is significantly higher in people over age 55 compared to younger people.[1] Of course, there's more than water to talk about when it comes to fluid intake. In this chapter, we tackle sugary drinks—and alcohol, too.

How Much Fluid Do You Need?

Some women are avid hydrators, carrying around water bottles wherever they go. But many women don't drink enough, either because they're busy and forget to drink, don't want to pee a lot, or simply don't get thirsty. Experts say women need about 9 cups of fluid daily from all sources. Some women may function fine with less, so consider 9 cups a general guide. Situations that drive fluid needs higher are exercising, particularly in hot weather, living in a hot environment, or dealing with an illness that increases fluid losses through fever, diarrhea, or vomiting.[2]

You know you're getting enough fluid when your pee is light yellow or clear. Signs of underhydration are more severe based on the degree of dehydration, but general signs include:[3]

- Thirst
- Dry mouth
- Less urination and darker urine
- Fatigue
- Headache
- Dizziness

Where to Find Fluid

Drinking water for hydration is great, but you don't have to rely solely on plain water to meet fluid needs. Fluid is found in fruits and vegetables, and in beverages other than water. Coffee, tea, herbal teas, milk, plain or flavored seltzer, and artificially sweetened beverages (our sweetener preference is stevia) also supply fluid, and we consider them healthy choices.[4]

Although coffee and tea contain caffeine, studies suggest they are not dehydrating when consumed in moderation.[5] Regular coffee drinking, including decaffeinated coffee, may actually reduce your risk of cardiovascular disease, type 2 diabetes, Parkinson's disease, and some cancers.[6] Tea drinkers benefit, too! Tea (particularly green tea) contains potent antioxidants called poly-phenols that may offer protection against cancer, diabetes, and cardiovascular and neurologic diseases.[7]

SOFT DRINKS WITH HARD CONSEQUENCES

Sipping too many sugar-sweetened beverages (SSBs) has health implications. SSBs contain added caloric sweeteners like sucrose (sugar), high-fructose corn syrup, or fruit juice concentrates, all of which have similar metabolic effects on the body. SSBs include a huge array of beverages, including coffeehouse concoctions with whipped cream and flavor shots, carbonated soft drinks, fruit drinks, sports drinks, energy and vitamin water drinks, sweetened teas, and "fruitades," which collectively are the largest contributors of added sugar intake in the United States.[8]

Bottled fruit and vegetable smoothies are touted as healthy, but most store-bought versions are loaded with sugar. Even many "green" and protein-rich smoothies average around 40 grams of carbohydrate per bottle, which is the equivalent of 10 level tea-spoons of sugar, and all-fruit versions may contain far more. Homemade protein smoothies are a great alternative. Check out our Peanut Butter Smoothie (page 257) and other "sensational smoothie" tips in chapter 12.

In recent decades, SSBs have closely paralleled the upsurge in obesity worldwide. And, while we can't say SSBs are entirely re-sponsible for excess weight, they aren't completely innocent, ei-ther. High intakes of SSBs are associated with weight gain and obesity, and can add an overwhelming number of calories to your day if you're not careful. The 250 calories from a 20-ounce soda or 15-ounce store-bought fruit smoothie, or the 300 to 500 calories in a 16-ounce sugary coffee drink, can tally up quickly, all while adding little to no nutritional value. It's thought that SSBs contribute to weight gain in part by making it easy to consume more calories without adding to our sense of fullness. In addition to any increased risk from weight gain alone, a steady intake of SSBs may raise the chances of type 2 diabetes and cardiovascular disease by stoking inflammation in the body, worsening insulin resistance, and damaging insulin-producing beta cells in the pancreas. Added sugars may also encourage belly fat accumulation, a common side effect of menopause, and contribute to high blood pressure, which tends to creep up with age.[9]

A recent large review of over 6,300 men and women found a significant association between SSBs and non-alcoholic fatty liver disease (NAFLD).[10] And even moderate amounts of SSBs cause problems.[11] Another study of over 2,600 middle-aged men and women found a higher prevalence of NAFLD among people who reported consuming more than one sugar-sweetened beverage daily compared to those who drank none, while no association was found with diet drinks.[12] The study's authors recommend reserving SSBs intake for special occasions. We could not agree more.

ALCOHOL: THE PROS AND CONS OF DRINKING

Many of us enjoy a tasty cocktail, a cold brew, or a glass of wine. If consumed in moderation, alcohol can be part of a healthy diet, but excess alcohol intake poses health hazards.

First, here are the pros about alcohol. A routine of light or moderate alcohol consumption, which is less than or equal to one drink a day for women and no more than two drinks per day for men, is associated with a lower risk of dying from any cause, coronary artery disease, type 2 diabetes, heart failure, and stroke.[13] However, the calories from alcohol must be factored into your daily calorie budget, according to the 2015–2020 Dietary Guidelines for Americans (DGA). Like nearly all SSBs, alcohol itself provides no nutrients, except for calories. The guidelines also say that if you don't drink, don't start doing so for health reasons.[14] It's also important to remember, as mentioned in chapter 6, no amount of alcohol is considered safe for preventing breast cancer.

Adhering to moderate alcohol consumption requires clarity on what constitutes a drink, and your idea of a drink may be very different from those of the experts! Examples of one drink include:

- Beer (5% alcohol): 12 fluid ounces
- Wine (12% alcohol): 5 fluid ounces
- Distilled spirits, such as rum, gin, vodka, and whisky (80-proof, 40% alcohol): 1.5 fluid ounces

Anything more than one drink per day is beyond moderation for women, and, no, you can't save up all your drinks for the weekend!

AND NOW FOR THE BAD NEWS

While moderate alcohol use may offer some health benefits, heavy drinking—including binge drinking—has no health benefits and can be harmful. Although men are more likely to overindulge than women, differences in body composition and chemistry cause women to absorb more alcohol. Plus, it takes a woman's body longer to break down alcohol and remove its by-products. This means alcohol hits women quicker and, its effects last longer. These differences also make it easier for excessive drinking to cause long-term health problems in women compared to men.[15] Some women may find alcohol aggravates their hot flashes, but there is no definitive research on the connection. Generally speaking, alcohol can interfere with sleep quality, which is already a challenge for many menopausal women.

What Works for Us

I just can't handle alcohol like I used to, and I particularly hate the dried-out feeling I sometimes get in the morning. To keep my drink intake to one (or two on special occasions), I always have seltzer water with lemon or lime after an alcoholic beverage. It still looks festive but provides the hydration I need, and it's an alternative to mindlessly reaching for another glass of wine.

—Hillary

Heavy drinking is defined as eight drinks or more per week for women. Binge drinking for women is defined as four or more drinks within two hours. According to the CDC, approximately 46% of adult women report drinking alcohol in the last thirty days, and 12% report binging three times per month, averaging five drinks per binge. They also identify the following concerns as specific to women who overindulge:[16]

- **Liver disease:** The risk of cirrhosis and other alcohol-related liver diseases is higher for women than for men.

- **Impact on the brain:** Excessive drinking may result in memory loss and shrinkage of the brain, and research suggests that women are more vulnerable. Damage also tends to appear with shorter periods of excessive drinking for women than for men.
- **Impact on the heart:** Studies show that women who drink excessively are at greater risk for heart damage than men, even when drinking at lower levels.
- **Cancer risk:** Alcohol consumption increases the risk of cancer of the mouth, throat, esophagus, liver, colon, and breast among women. Breast cancer risk rises as alcohol use increases.

Studies show that women are 70% more likely to experience depression than men, and twice as likely to develop an anxiety disorder, particularly during the menopause transition. Both conditions can be triggers for using alcohol as a means of coping with mental health stress.[17] Unfortunately, a recent study shows that problem drinking is on the rise among women and older adults in general.[18] The study examined how drinking patterns changed between 2002 and 2013, based on in-person surveys of tens of thousands of U.S. adults. The results show a narrowing of the "gender gap" in drinking disorders. Though men are still more likely than women to be problem drinkers, women are catching up, which may be due to stress and a greater acceptance of alcohol consumption by women.

The Warning Signs of Drinking Too Much

There are an estimated 15 million alcohol abusers in the United States, and about 4.6 million of them are women.[19] Signs and symptoms of alcohol abuse may include spending a lot of time drinking or recovering from alcohol use, wanting to cut down on how much you drink but being unsuccessful, or continuing to drink alcohol even though you know it's causing physical, social, or interpersonal problems. A more extensive list of symptoms that could suggest alcohol abuse disorder can be found on the National Institute of Alcohol Abuse and Alcoholism website.[20] If you suspect you may have an alcohol use problem for any reason, please confide in a health professional or counselor who can help you find the support you need.

What to Drink Instead of Alcohol

If you've decided to limit or avoid alcohol, it's often helpful to have alcohol-free alternatives, especially in social situations, where people may prod you to drink. To avoid replacing alcohol with sugary drinks, check out these five lower-calorie "mocktails":

- Club soda or carbonated mineral water and a splash of 100% juice

- Iced green or black tea
- Coconut water
- Maple water
- Fruit-infused water (add sliced lemon, lime, orange, or grape-fruit, or sliced berries to a pitcher of water; let sit for a few hours in the refrigerator and enjoy)

Medications and Alcohol

The potential dangers of alcohol's interacting with medication are real and should be taken very seriously. Mixing alcohol with certain drugs can cause nausea and vomiting, headaches, drowsiness, fainting, or loss of coordination. It also can put you at risk for internal bleeding, heart problems, and difficulty breathing. Alcohol can also make medications less effective or useless, or it may make the medication toxic to your body. Combining medications with herbal remedies may also produce harmful effects.[21]

Older people are at increased risk of alcohol/medication interactions, and hundreds of common prescription and over-the-counter drugs may cause harmful interactions, including certain heart and diabetes medications, non-steroidal anti-inflammatories (like ibuprofen and naproxen), acetaminophen, and blood thinners. If you're not sure if your medications can be combined with alcohol, ask your doctor or pharmacist if it's safe.

Calculating Alcohol Calories

The calories in wine, beer, and other alcoholic beverages can really add up, and mixed drinks are the worst. Everyone mixes cocktails differently, but here are some calorie estimates for cocktails and other boozy beverages:

DRINK	NUMBER OF CALORIES
Margarita	300
Martini	241
Cosmopolitan	227
Beer, higher-alcohol (12 ounces)	209
Beer (12 ounces)	192
Vodka and tonic	189
Gin and tonic	189
Bloody Mary	155
Rum and diet cola	135
Vodka and soda	133
Red Zinfandel wine (5 ounces)	130
Chardonnay (5 ounces)	125

(continued)

DRINK	NUMBER OF CALORIES
Spiked seltzer, 5% alcohol (12 ounces)	110
Beer, light (12 ounces)	103
80-proof rum, gin, vodka, or whiskey (1.5 ounces)	96

Source: U.S. Department of Agriculture, Agricultural Research Service, U.S.D.A. Food Composition Databases; available at https://ndb.nal.usda.gov/ndb/.

9

LET'S GET PHYSICAL!

I know exercise is important for a lot of reasons, but it can be a challenge to get enough with my busy schedule.

—*Noreen, age 48*

What helps counteract the effects of menopause and is effective in any amount? Exercise, of course! Of all the healthy lifestyle habits to develop and maintain, regular exercise is one of the best, no matter your age, body weight, or health issues. Physical activity is particularly vital after age 40, when it helps to offset the effects of hormonal changes and naturally improves health and happiness.

You don't have to love exercise, and it's okay if you simply tolerate it as another item on your to-do list. We support all views about exercise except the idea that working out is punishment for your past or present diet or body weight. Now is the time to make regular exercise a part of your life. And by now, we mean today. Exercise offers instant rewards and long-lasting benefits, including a better mood, a chance to socialize, and fun.

Most of us spend the majority of our waking hours sitting or reclining. Long commutes and desk jobs necessitate such sedentary behavior. However, extended periods of inactivity on a consistent basis increase the risk for dying early from all causes, including cardiovascular disease, type 2 diabetes, and colon, endometrial, and lung cancers.

Here's the good news: No matter how sedentary you are, gradually increasing moderate-intensity physical activity helps to improve health. A 2019 observational study of women ages 63 to 97 found that reducing sedentary time by an hour a day was linked to a 12% lower risk for cardiovascular disease and a 26% lower risk for developing heart disease over a period of five years.[1]

Move More for Your Life

The beauty of physical activity is that it starts improving your life right away, and if you keep it up, it will help safeguard your mental and physical health. It's difficult to ignore the therapeutic effects of exercise on mood, sleep, hot flashes, and so many other aspects of health of concern during the transition to menopause. Here's why exercise is an investment in your present and future well-being.

Preserves and builds skeletal muscle. Muscles attached to your skeleton move your body parts and hold your bones and joints in the most functional and least painful positions. Most of the tissue in the body is skeletal muscle, and it's worth preserving for many reasons, including protecting joints and internal organs, maintaining balance and coordination, and promoting overall health.[2]

Everyone starts to lose meaningful amounts of skeletal muscle around age 40, but declining estrogen levels in menopause accelerate the process and make it harder to produce new muscle.[3] Skeletal muscle is constantly being produced and broken down. Skeletal muscle stores amino acids, the building blocks of protein. The body requires a steady supply of amino acids to maintain normal levels in the blood, skin, brain, and heart and to produce glucose, the energy for cells. When blood levels of amino acids are low between meals, the body borrows from skeletal muscle. After you eat protein, the body repays muscle with amino acid deposits.

Skeletal muscle also stores glycogen, which is a source of energy for muscle cells, and utilizes most of the insulin in the body to store glycogen. A decline in muscle tissue may contribute to insulin resistance or make it worse, which could result in type 2 diabetes and other health problems.[4]

Skeletal muscle burns more calories than fat, 24/7. The opposite is also true—losing muscle reduces metabolic rate, making it more difficult to control your weight.

Estrogen protects skeletal muscle by helping to reduce inflammation that may lead to loss of muscle mass, strength, and function.[5] As estrogen levels drop, there's an increase in muscle tissue loss and fat accumulation in muscle tissue. Exercise helps protect muscles by preventing fat deposition within skeletal muscle.[6] In addition, menopausal belly fat worsens the problem by causing inflammation that contributes to the breakdown of muscle.

Some loss of skeletal muscle mass and strength is unavoidable with age and menopause, but of all the reasons for the decline, inactivity takes the cake. It's likely that regular exercise alters muscles so that they become better at building muscle cells.[7]

Nutrition plays a starring role in making and preserving skeletal muscle before, during, and after menopause. See page 173 for a discussion on what to eat to support muscle health.

Reduces the risk for heart disease and stroke. Exercise helps to lower blood pressure, triglycerides (fat), and LDL ("bad") cholesterol in the blood, and it raises HDL ("good") cholesterol. Aerobic activity, including walking, biking, and swimming, improves circulation and strengthens heart and lung function, and is linked to a reduced risk for heart disease and stroke. Regular aerobic exercise also reduces inflammation, which encourages and worsens cardiovascular disease and other chronic conditions, such as cancer, diabetes, and Alzheimer's disease. Exercise is so important to heart health that experts liken inactivity to having high blood pressure, high blood cholesterol, or smoking.[8]

Promotes a longer life. Strong scientific evidence shows that physical activity delays dying early from all causes. Experts estimate that people who are physically active for a total of about two and a half hours a week (150 minutes) have a much lower risk of dying early than those who are sedentary (inactive), and the risk declines with increasing activity. The best part is that any physical activity produces health benefits.[9]

Improves sleep. Sleep problems are a huge issue for menopausal women, and those who are regularly physically active may sleep better and feel well rested. Moderate and vigorous physical activity are associated with an easier time falling asleep, more time spent sleeping, a better quality of sleep, less daytime sleepiness, and using fewer sleep-aid medications. People with insomnia and obstructive sleep apnea may also benefit from regular exercise.[10]

Anatomy of a Hot Flash

A hot flash is the sudden onset of heat that seems to come out of nowhere, causing flushing and sweating. Hot flashes last from about 1 to 5 minutes but can feel like an eternity, especially when they are particularly intense. Experts say that hot flashes are a result of a fluctuation in hormone levels that affect the part of the brain that regulates body temperature—your internal thermostat, of sorts. The brain becomes hypersensitive to even minor increases in the temperature of the air around you and starts to overreact to cool you down. Blood flows away from the core of your body and your brain and goes to the blood vessels in your skin, which open up and make you feel hot. You then start sweating profusely to help bring down your core temperature. As sweat evaporates from your skin, it takes some body heat with it.

Night sweats are repeated episodes of extreme perspiration that may soak your PJs and bedding. If you are around age 50 and have irregular or absent menstrual periods, night sweats are hot flashes that happen at night. However, if night sweats are accompanied by a fever, weight loss, localized pain, cough, diarrhea, or other symptoms of concern, talk with your doctor or nurse practitioner. Certain medications can also cause night sweats.[11]

May ease hot flashes. Hot flashes and trouble sleeping, which often go hand in hand, are the biggest problems associated with menopause. Hot flashes won't hurt you, but they can be irritating and even debilitating, depending on their frequency and severity. Having hot flashes at work, when you're out, or during the night can be nerve-racking. Hot flashes can make it difficult to get enough quality sleep, which can diminish energy and productivity during the day.

About 80% of women living in the United States experience hot flashes. African American women tend to have the most severe and persistent hot flashes, while Asian Americans in the United States report the fewest. Some women have hot flashes in their 40s and 50s, when they are still having menstrual cycles, while others start having hot flashes only when their cycles have stopped. Hot flashes can last for upwards of seven years, and for some they can be quite severe and unpredictable.[12]

Exercise may provide some relief from hot flashes. Sixteen weeks of supervised regular aerobic exercise of moderate intensity in postmenopausal women with hot flashes reduced the flow of blood to the skin and sweating and improved blood flow to the brain during hot flashes.[13]

A 2019 study found that a fifteen-week weight-training regimen helped fight hot flashes in postmenopausal women, none of whom had exercised regularly before the study. Women in the exercise group had about half as many hot flashes as those who made no changes to their physical activity, and the flashes were less severe in intensity.[14]

Higher levels of lower-intensity physical activity may also help women with hot flashes sleep better and wake up less often during the night. Research shows that even working around the house or doing other light activities may yield benefits when you hit the hay.[15]

How to Handle Hot Flashes

The most effective management of hot flashes is with hormone replacement therapy (HRT), but it's not right for every woman. Speak with your doctor or nurse practitioner about whether HRT or another prescription medication is a good idea for you. Other than getting regular exercise, dressing in layers, and avoiding warm rooms and hot drinks, here are some strategies to help minimize hot flash symptoms:[16]

- Cognitive behavioral therapy (CBT) is a type of talk therapy that may help decrease the symptoms of hot flashes in healthy postmenopausal women and breast cancer survivors. CBT may also help with your mood, sleep, and quality of life.
- Relaxation therapy, which may have a small effect.
- Acupuncture. Research shows that acupuncture can reduce hot flashes in healthy perimenopausal and menopausal women.
- Stopping smoking. Smoking is a known risk factor for hot flashes, and quitting may help reduce the symptoms.[17]

Lowers type 2 diabetes risk. Regular physical activity reduces the chance for type 2 diabetes in every adult, no matter her body weight, and it's also vital for managing the condition. Exercise promotes glucose uptake by muscles, and regular physical activity appears to condition muscle cells to improve their sensitivity to insulin, which reduces the amount of insulin the pancreas must produce to regulate blood glucose.[18]

Regular aerobic exercise and strength-training activities both work to improve blood glucose control. In a recent analysis that included 360 older people with type 2 diabetes, resistance training for at least eight weeks was linked to improved muscle strength and long-term decreases in blood glucose levels.[19]

Reduces cancer risk. Regular exercise is one of many lifestyle factors known to reduce the risk for certain types of cancer and may improve survival.[20] See chapter 6 for more on the relationship between exercise and cancer risk.

Encourages better brain function. All older adults, even the healthiest of us, experience some cognitive decline. We don't process information as quickly, our memory isn't quite as sharp, and our ability to plan, organize, and control our emotions—considered executive functions—wane a bit. Exercise can help.

Studies show that compared to inactive people, those who do greater amounts of moderate- or vigorous-intensity exercise perform better on tests of academic achievement and neuropsychological health, such as those involving mental processing speed, memory, and other executive functions.

Physical activity also helps to ward off cognitive impairment, which occurs when a person has trouble remembering, learning, concentrating, or making decisions that affect his or her everyday life. A 2019 study found that a single 30-minute session of moderate-intensity aerobic exercise improved memory in healthy older adults ages 55 to 85 years by activating the hippocampus, the part of the brain associated with memory that is attacked first in Alzheimer's disease.[21] Other research shows regular aerobic exercise (twice weekly for six months) increased the volume of the hippocampus, which gradually shrinks with age, in older women. In theory, a greater brain volume may delay the onset of illnesses such as Alzheimer's.[22]

Low-intensity activity is also tied to brain health. In a 2019 study, researchers found that every additional hour of low-intensity physical activity was linked to greater brain volume in midlife adults even when they did less than the suggested amount of exercise, which could mean physical activity has the potential for preventing dementia.[23]

Reduces symptoms of depression and anxiety. Regular exercise may lower the risk of depression and make anxiety easier to manage, and it may help control mood swings during perimenopause and menopause.

Working out reduces levels of adrenaline and cortisol—hormones the body makes in excess when you're feeling stressed. Physical activity also stimulates the production of feel-good compounds such as anandamide and serotonin, which travel to the brain and help ward off symptoms of anxiety and depression.[24] A 2019 study found that replacing 15 minutes of sitting with 15 minutes of running, or swapping 1 hour of sitting with 1 hour of moderate activity like brisk walking, boosted mood. Any kind of movement, including taking the stairs instead of the elevator, contributed to depression prevention.[25]

Promotes bone health. Menopause is hard on bones. Declining estrogen levels weaken bones and make them more prone to fracture. Exercise helps counteract some of these effects by slowing the loss of bone tissue.

Protects joints. Estrogen loss may be involved in the development of osteoarthritis (OA). In OA, the cartilage in joints wears down, resulting in joint pain and damage. Regular, moderate-intensity physical activity may help women with OA before and after menopause.[26]

Improves the gut microbiome. In a recent study, non-exercisers gradually increased their physical activity to an hour of vigorous jogging or pedaling three times a week. This increased activity was associated with a bump in the number of beneficial gut bacteria that produce short-chain fatty acids—compounds that help reduce inflammation and improve insulin resistance. When researchers again measured the participants' gut microbes six weeks after stopping exercise completely, their guts had returned to their original composition, suggesting that regular exercise may be key to a better gut microbiome.[27]

Take Exercise One Session at a Time

Exercise provides instant gratification. According to the Physical Activity Guidelines for Americans (PAG), a single session of moderate to vigorous physical activity, such as a brisk 30-minute walk or a challenging weights class, can immediately reduce blood pressure, improve insulin sensitivity and sleep (on the same day as the exercise), reduce anxiety symptoms, and improve certain brain functions. Even better, the health benefits of physical activity have nothing to do with your weight. Everyone wins!

Helps with weight control. Regular exercise can slow or reduce weight gain and help promote weight loss, particularly when it's paired with a balanced eating plan. Many women need more than 150 minutes (2½ hours) of moderate-intensity activity a week (or the equivalent) to maintain their weight; those aiming to lose or maintain a substantial weight loss may need double that amount. Increasing your physical activity helps reduce belly fat, which lowers the risk for cardiovascular disease and other health problems.[28]

What Type of Exercise and How Much Do You Need?

Working out is a must for battling midlife weight gain, but not if you rely on it to torch the calories in a pint of fatty ice cream, a half bag of snack chips, or that extra cocktail. Most people think their workouts burn more calories than they do (our hands are raised!), and it's easy to overcompensate with food, particularly if your workouts are vigorous. Find a combination of activities that raises your heart rate and strengthens muscles without triggering intense hunger.

AEROBIC ACTIVITY

Aerobic activity, such as brisk walking, singles tennis, and power yoga, is the kind that makes your heart beat faster and your lungs work harder. In addition to intensity, frequency and duration matter for aerobic activity. Adults who do the equivalent of at least 150 minutes (2½ hours) to 300 minutes (5 hours, total) of moderate-intensity aerobic activity each week gain substantial health benefits, described earlier in this chapter.

Generally speaking, vigorous-intensity activity is twice as difficult as moderate-intensity. That means runners and other vigorous exercisers need a minimum of 75 minutes (1¼ hours) to 150 minutes (2½ hours) of exercise weekly to meet the suggested exercise guidelines, while brisk walkers need at least 150 minutes (2½ hours) to 300 minutes (5 hours) worth of exercise every week. Doing more than the minimum yields additional benefits. For example, exercising for a total of 300 minutes a week is associated with an even lower risk of heart disease or type 2 diabetes than 150 minutes a week.[29]

It's best to exercise for at least 30 minutes on five different days. However, the total amount of moderate-to-vigorous physical activity you do is more important than the length of each exercise episode, so fit in workouts whenever you can.

Moderate- and Vigorous-Intensity Activities

Exercise intensity is relative. For example, if you're just getting back to exercise, moderate-intensity activities may feel vigorous to you. Or, you may find moderate-intensity activities aren't challenging.

To determine intensity, the "talk test" will help you to exercise at a pace that you can maintain. You should be able to talk, but not sing, during an aerobic activity that's of moderate-intensity for you. If you cannot say more than a few words without pausing for a breath, that activity is of vigorous-intensity for you.

MODERATE-INTENSITY ACTIVITIES
Walking briskly (2.5 mph per hour or faster)
Recreational swimming

Bicycling slower than 10 mph on level terrain

Tennis (doubles)

Active forms of yoga (for example, Vinyasa or
power yoga*)

Ballroom or line dancing

General yard and home repair work

Exercise classes such as water aerobics

VIGOROUS-INTENSITY ACTIVITIES

Jogging or running

Swimming laps

Tennis (singles)

Vigorous dancing

Bicycling faster than 10 mph

Jumping rope

Heavy yard work (digging or shoveling, with heart
rate increases)

Hiking uphill or with a heavy backpack

Exercise classes like kickboxing or vigorous step
aerobics

Power yoga

High-intensity interval training (HIIT), a form of
interval training that consists of alternating short
periods of maximal-effort exercise with lower-
intensity recovery periods

*According to the PAG, yoga may include time that would be counted as light-intensity physical activity or as moderate-intensity physical activity. Yoga may also be considered an aerobic and muscle-strengthening activity, depending on the type and the postures practiced. Tai chi is typically a light-intensity physical activity but may be considered moderate-intensity for some adults. Tai chi involves balance activities, and some forms of tai chi can strengthen muscles.

MUSCLE-STRENGTHENING ACTIVITIES

In addition to aerobic activity, the PAG suggests doing muscle-strengthening activities of moderate or greater intensity. Muscle-strengthening activity, including resistance training and weight lifting, forces muscles to work or hold against an applied force. You can also strengthen muscles using your body weight, such as doing push-ups, pull-ups, and planks.

Muscle-strengthening activities bolster bones and improve skeletal muscle mass, strength, and function, and they help maintain muscle mass, particularly during weight loss. A 2019 review notes that regular resistance exercise also helps prevent type 2 diabetes, cardiovascular disease, cancer, and mobility issues as we age.[30]

For the greatest good, resistance training should overload the major muscle groups of the body, which include the legs, hips, back, chest, abdomen, shoulders, and arms, on at least two days of every week. Perform muscle-strengthening exercises to the point where you think it would be difficult to do another repetition. One set of 8 to 12 repetitions of each exercise is effective to enhance strength, although two or three sets is likely more effective, especially as you become stronger. Improvements in muscle strength and endurance will progress with time as long as you gradually increase the amount of weight or resistance, the days a week of you spend on resistance activities, or both.[31]

What Works for Us

In my 20s and 30s, running dominated my workout regimen, and strength training was an afterthought. To be honest, I was eager to control my weight and I thought that aerobic exercise was the way to go. That all changed in my 40s, when I began to realize the many benefits of lifting weights and other resistance exercise. I still run and take kickboxing classes, but strength training now plays an equal role in my exercise routine.

—Liz

All Movement Matters

Standing on one leg or using a wobble board while working out is a great way to work on balance. Flexibility activities, such as stretching, help preserve and enhance the ability of joints to move through the full range of motion. Although time spent doing balance and flexibility activities does not count toward meeting PAG exercise guidelines, they may help reduce injury. Bone-strengthening activities, such as such as jumping jacks, running, brisk walking, and weight lifting, can double as aerobic and muscle-strengthening activities.

HOW TO START EXERCISING AGAIN

You may have spent the last decade—or two—with little time or motivation (or both) to work out. Here's what to consider before you start exercising again.

Get good advice. In general, healthy people who plan gradual increases in their physical activity do not need to consult a healthcare provider unless they have a chronic health problem or disability. If you're unsure about exercise, seek instruction from a certified personal trainer who understands midlife women and won't push you to do too much too soon.

Avoid injury. Creating a small overload on muscles, joints, and bones, and waiting for the body to adapt and recover reduces injury risk. You've overdone it when your muscles stay sore for more than a few days after working out.

Take baby steps. When it comes to movement, any is better than none. Small increases in moderate-intensity physical activity provide health benefits, even if you've been sedentary for years, or your exercise has been spotty. Walking is free and easy and can be done just about anywhere. Start by walking 5 minutes several times each day for five or six days a week. Gradually increase the walking time to 10 minutes a session, three times daily, and slowly increase your speed so that you cover more ground.

Be realistic. Approach your workouts from where you are now, not where you used to be or want to be. Your body is different from when you were 30 years old, and chances are you can't do the workouts you did before. (For example, we avoid activities that involve a lot of jumping because we've each had three children!)

Whatever you do, don't wait to become more active. Feel good about increasing your physical activity, no matter by how much. Take heart in knowing that simply sitting less is good for your health.

HOW TO STAY MOTIVATED TO EXERCISE

When you're in a long-term relationship with exercise, maintaining momentum can be challenging. Though we both enjoy exercise, we still have days when we drag ourselves to the gym because we're tired or would prefer to do something else. Unexpected life events have ruined our best-laid exercise plans more times than we can count. Our advice: Be persistent. Here's how we deal with common exercise barriers.

Make it fun. You're more likely to stay active if you choose enjoyable activities, not what you think you should do. Try something new, such as yoga, Pilates, water aerobics, or aerial fitness. If you're not a gym person, take up (or return to) tennis or golf, or spend an hour at the driving range or hiking.

Multitask. Listen to an audiobook, music, or a podcast when you walk, run, or bike. Lift weights, use resistance bands, or walk the treadmill while you watch your favorite show.

Find a friend. Exercising with others is motivating and increases accountability. Women who are physically active on a consistent basis are more likely to have a "buddy" who is also active.[32] Stroll or hike with a friend before sharing a meal. Meet up with an office mate for a walk after lunch. Join a spinning or yoga class with a group of friends.

Always have a Plan B. Can't run outside because it's too hot, cold, or rainy? Join a gym and use the treadmill. Can't make it to class? Take one online or on cable TV. Invest in a set of weights and bands for when you can't get to the gym. Always pack a pair of comfortable walking shoes so that you can walk anywhere, at any time. Forgot your gym bag? Leave a bag with exercise clothes in your trunk.

Shake it up. Bored? Add variety. For example, if you run five days a week, cut back to three and swap in kickboxing classes or swimming. Balance higher-intensity workouts, such as singles tennis, with more moderate ones.

Schedule workouts. Block time to exercise and treat working out like an important client, friend, or family member. There will be times when you cannot get to the gym or stay for as long as you want, and that's okay.

Set exercise goals. Vowing to "work out more" is vague. Set measurable exercise goals to better stay on track, like walking three times a week on specific days for 50 minutes each time.

Substitute. Pressed for time? Swap some moderate-intensity activity for the vigorous-intensity kind. Use the 2-to-1 rule of thumb: 15 minutes of vigorous-intensity aerobic activity is as beneficial as 30 minutes of moderate-intensity exercise. For example, instead of walking for 40 minutes, run for 20.

Just keep moving. Commit to maintaining *some* type of activity no matter how busy you get or how little you want to work out.

Dress the part. When your motivation has really tanked, try changing into your workout clothes and lacing up your sneakers. The thought of changing again without working out may be just the motivation you need to get up and go!

The Power of Protein

Regular exercise, particularly the strength-training type, is critical for maximizing skeletal muscle during the menopausal transition, and after. Your body also needs adequate protein as part of a balanced eating plan.

Protein and physical activity are a dynamic duo. Together, they prompt the body to produce more skeletal muscle than either can make on their own. Protein is part of every cell in our body and can be used for energy, if necessary. A balanced diet with adequate carbohydrate for energy prevents protein from being used for its calories.

After digestion, protein from food is released into the bloodstream as amino acids, which prompts muscle cell production and halts its breakdown. As we age, it's harder for our body to make muscle, even in the presence of adequate levels of amino acids.[33] Losing estrogen compounds this effect. Though it's more difficult to make and keep muscle after menopause, it's possible with the right mix of exercise and good nutrition, particularly protein.

HOW MUCH PROTEIN DO YOU NEED?

The Recommended Dietary Allowance (RDA) is based on body weight: 0.8 grams of protein per kilogram of body weight per day, which is equal to 0.36 grams of protein per pound per day. That means a 150-pound (68-kilogram) woman requires 59 grams of protein daily.[34] (To get your body weight in kilograms, divide it by 2.2.)

A growing body of literature suggests that the current protein RDA may not be sufficient to optimize muscle health, expecially in people over age 50. Experts argue that while the protein RDA prevents deficiencies, it's unlikely that it supports the maintenance of muscle tissue. In addition, the RDA doesn't account for research showing that while older people are capable of making as much muscle as younger individuals, they require more protein to achieve the same effect.[35]

The European Society for Clinical and Economic Aspects of Osteoporosis, Osteoarthritis, and Musculoskeletal Diseases (ESCEO) recommends women over age 50 consume 1.0 to 1.2 grams of protein per kilogram of body weight daily in conjunction with regular exercise to prevent the loss of muscle mass, strength, and bone. For a 150-pound woman, they suggest 68 to 81 grams of protein daily, or about 23 grams more protein per day than the RDA.[36]

In an observational study of nearly 400 women ages 60 to 90, researchers found that consuming an average of 1.1 grams of protein per kilogram per day was associated with less body fat and greater muscle strength than eating less than 0.8 grams per kilogram per day.[37]

The Menopause Diet Plan accounts for these higher protein recommendations, as you'll see in the meal plans.

WHY PROTEIN QUALITY MATTERS

The amount and quality of protein you eat matters. Animal and plant foods both provide amino acids, but the protein in animal foods, such as lean meat, poultry, eggs, dairy, and seafood, is different from nearly every plant source.

Animal foods supply all the amino acids that the body cannot produce, known as indispensable amino acids (IAAs) and sometimes called essential amino acids (EAAs). You need to get IAAs from food. With the exception of soy, quinoa, and buckwheat, nearly all plant foods lack adequate amounts of IAAs. Consistently coming up short on IAAs can limit muscle mass and strength and have other effects on overall health in menopausal women.

Though animal and plant proteins can provide the required essential amino acids for health, animal proteins typically have more leucine, the only amino acid that triggers the muscle-making process. Leucine is the focus of ongoing research, and it's possible that older adults require more leucine to stimulate muscle tissue production at rest and after resistance exercise.[38, 39]

In a study of women and men ages 35 to 65, consuming about 7 grams a day of leucine along with adequate protein was linked to keeping more lean body mass over a period of six years.[40] This chart will help you get the protein and leucine you need.

FOOD TYPE	PROTEIN (GRAMS)	LEUCINE (GRAMS)
Chicken breast, boneless, skinless (4 ounces), cooked	36	2.7
Tuna, canned, drained (4 ounces)	33	1.7
Pork tenderloin (4 ounces), roasted	29	2.7
Shrimp (4 ounces), cooked	26	2.2

FOOD TYPE	PROTEIN (GRAMS)	LEUCINE (GRAMS)
Tempeh (4 ounces), cooked	26	NA
Beef, ground, 95% lean (4 ounces), cooked	25	2.0
Haddock (4 ounces), cooked	23	2.1
Yogurt, Greek, plain, non-fat (1 cup)	22	2.2
Tofu, firm (4 ounces)	13	0.9
Cottage cheese, low-fat (½ cup)	12	1.4
Yogurt, plain, low-fat (8 ounces)	11	1.2
Lentils (½ cup), cooked	9	0.65
Peanut butter (2 tablespoons)	9	0.5
Peanuts (¼ cup)	9	0.6
Milk, 1% low-fat (1 cup)	8	0.8

Milk, whole (1 cup)	8	0.8
Soybeans (edamame) (¼ cup), dry roasted	8	0.75
Soy beverage (1 cup)	7	0.45
Black beans, canned, drained (½ cup)	7	0.6
Almond butter (2 tablespoons)	6	0.5
Almonds, whole, 23 nuts (¼ cup)	6	0.4
Cheddar cheese (1 ounce)	6	0.63
Egg (1 large)	6	0.55
Pistachios, shelled (¼ cup)	6	0.5
Walnuts, chopped (¼ cup)	5	0.3
Garbanzo beans, canned, drained (½ cup)	4	0.15
Quinoa (½ cup), cooked	4	0.25
Buckwheat (½ cup), cooked	3	0.15

(continued)

FOOD TYPE	PROTEIN (GRAMS)	LEUCINE (GRAMS)
Corn (½ cup), cooked	3	0.55

Source: U.S. Department of Agriculture, Agricultural Research Service, U.S.D.A. Food Composition Databases; available at https://ndb.nal .usda.gov/ndb/.

DO YOU NEED PROTEIN POWDER?

Protein powders are concentrated sources of protein. They're made from animal or plant foods, such as dairy, soybeans, and peas. Though we don't suggest using them as replacements for protein-rich foods, protein powders can help you more easily meet your protein and leucine needs.

Whey protein powder is derived from cow's milk, has all the amino acids to make proteins in the body, and is rich in leucine. It's also digested quickly. Soy protein powder has all the essential amino acids, but less leucine than whey, and it's absorbed more slowly. Pea protein powder has a bit less leucine than soy, but unlike soy, it does not contain all the essential amino acids. Pea protein powder shows promise, and we look forward to more research about its efficacy.

Adding more protein to your eating plan adds calories that you must account for, and you should do resistance training at least twice weekly to maximize the effects of dietary protein.

WHEN TO EAT PROTEIN

Skeletal muscle tissue is in a constant state of flux so it's important to "feed" it at every meal. However, most of us skimp on protein at breakfast, do only slightly better at lunch, and eat the majority of our protein at dinner, which is less than ideal for preserving muscle. Studies suggest an even distribution of protein throughout the day helps maximize muscle-making by the body, especially when combined with physical activity.[41]

In one study of premenopausal women and men, those who consumed 30 grams of protein at each of three meals made 25% more muscle over a 24-hour period compared to people who ate the same amount of protein but most of it in the evening.[42]

Though more research on protein timing is needed, especially in perimenopausal and menopausal women, it won't hurt to eat protein and leucine at regular intervals throughout the day as part of a balanced diet. ESCEO recommends women consume 20 to 25 grams of protein at every meal, in conjunction with regular resistance training exercise.[43]

The Menopause Diet Plan will help you get enough protein at every meal and snack, and includes many leucine-rich food choices.

What Works for Us

Whey protein powder recently became a daily part of my eating plan as a direct result of researching this book. As I learned about the benefits of consuming protein for menopausal women, I started using half a scoop of whey protein at breakfast to help me get a total of 25 grams of protein for the meal. While I prefer whole foods, it's not realistic for me to expect to get the protein I need in the morning from food alone.

—Liz

Beyond Protein:
Other Factors in Muscle Health

There are several other considerations affecting muscle health, including the following.

VITAMIN D

Vitamin D appears to enhance the effect of protein on muscle cell production, and it plays a key role in muscle function, too. We make less vitamin D as we age, and we absorb less from the digestive tract. See chapter 7 for more about vitamin D needs.

OMEGA-3 FATS

Omega-3 fats, found naturally in seafood and added to other foods, support muscle mass, strength, and function.[44] In one study, a group of women with an average age of 64 who took 2,000 milligrams of fish oil daily and did resistance exercise for a 90-day period improved their muscle strength as compared to women who exercised only.[45] Fish is also an excellent source of protein and leucine, as well as many other nutrients. Rather than taking large amounts of omega-3 supplements, we suggest including seafood at least two times a week.

STATIN DRUGS

People who take statin drugs, such as Lipitor, may experience mild muscle cramping, soreness, weakness, and fatigue. Women are especially prone to these muscle problems, and other side effects of statin drugs, which may be more likely to happen during or after strenuous bouts of exercise.[46]

10

ALL ABOUT DIETARY
SUPPLEMENTS

Entering menopause got me thinking more seriously
about my bones, so I figured it was a good time to get
more consistent with taking extra calcium and vitamin D.

—*Alison, age 59*

A balanced eating plan is the best strategy for getting the nutrients you need. However, it's probably impossible to eat
perfectly every day, and although many women have access
to relatively affordable food, the typical American diet bears little
resemblance to what experts recommend. In addition, menopause
and aging increase the need for several vitamins and minerals,
known as micronutrients. Though the Menopause Diet Plan includes a variety of foods, you may need dietary supplements based
on your choices.

About half of all adults in the United States take at least one micronutrient dietary supplement—more women than men. Before
popping supplements, including the botanical kind that women
may take to manage menopausal symptoms, there's a few things
you should know about this popular trend.[1]

How Age and Menopause Change Vitamin and Mineral Needs

Turning 50 influences your requirements for certain micronutrients, and so do perimenopause and menopause.

Calcium. Calcium supports the heart, muscles, and bones, among other parts of the body. The body absorbs less calcium from foods and dietary supplements with age, which jeopardizes bone health. To help combat age-related problems, a woman's calcium needs increase from 1,000 milligrams (mg) daily to 1,200 milligrams (mg) a day after age 50.[2]

Dairy foods are concentrated sources of calcium, and some, such as milk, have added vitamin D to promote calcium absorption. Women who limit or avoid dairy products may not get enough calcium at any age. Vitamin D needs don't change after age 50, but women should consume 600 International Units (IU) of vitamin D every day, and more if they've been diagnosed with a deficiency. Chapter 7 has information about calcium and vitamin D in foods.[3]

Vitamin B6. The need for vitamin B_6, which helps support energy metabolism and contributes to heart health, increases to 1.9 milligrams a day after age 50. Vitamin B_6 is found in animal and plant foods, including fish, chicken, and garbanzo beans, and it's also added to fortified grain foods, such as breakfast cereal, bread, and pasta. Vitamin B_6 is a water-soluble nutrient, which means the body doesn't store it and requires it every day. A balanced diet with a variety of foods helps to satisfy vitamin B_6 needs.[4]

Vitamin B$_{12}$. The many functions of vitamin B$_{12}$ include helping to produce red blood cells and DNA, and supporting heart and nervous system health. Vitamin B$_{12}$ needs don't change in women over 50, but the synthetic form is better absorbed at midlife and beyond.

Starting at age 14, females require 2.4 micrograms of vitamin B$_{12}$ daily. After age 50, women (and men) should rely on synthetic B$_{12}$, found in dietary supplements and foods with added vitamin B$_{12}$, such as fortified grains and nutritional yeast, to meet most of their needs. That's because older people produce less stomach acid and may absorb less natural B$_{12}$, found only in animal foods such as seafood, meat, milk, and eggs. Synthetic B$_{12}$ is processed without stomach acid, making it more available to the body. Foods naturally rich in B$_{12}$ should still be part of a nutritious eating plan.[5]

Iron. As part of red blood cells, iron is necessary to deliver oxygen to every cell, among other functions. Iron is found in animal and plant foods, including meat, seafood, and legumes, and it's added to fortified grains and dietary supplements. After age 50 (around the time of menopause), women's daily iron needs drop from 18 milligrams to 8 milligrams a day. In general, after menopause women should choose dietary supplements with little to no iron to prevent iron overload in the body, but should continue to consume iron-rich foods as part of a balanced diet.[6]

How Dietary Supplements
Are Regulated

Dietary supplements are regulated by the U.S. Food and Drug Administration (FDA), which also oversees the quality and safety of food and medications. The Dietary Supplement Health and Education Act of 1994 (DSHEA) defines and sets safety and labeling requirements for dietary supplements. However, dietary supplements are not regulated with the same scrutiny as medications.

The FDA is not required by law to review dietary supplements, unlike prescription and over-the-counter drugs, for safety and effectiveness before they are marketed. Instead, manufacturers and/or distributors of dietary supplements are responsible for ensuring product safety, including accurate labeling and keeping their products free from contaminants, such as bacteria, pesticides, and lead and other heavy metals. The FDA takes action against manufacturers if their products are found to be unsafe, adulterated, and/or misbranded (for example, if labeling is false or misleading) or if products marketed as dietary supplements are making claims to diagnose, manage, treat, cure, or prevent a disease.[7]

Most dietary supplements, especially multivitamins and single vitamin and mineral supplements produced by large, well-known companies, are high quality. ConsumerReports.com offers information about dietary supplement safety and quality, and independent organizations, such as ConsumerLab.com, test supplements, but there is usually a fee to access the information.

Why You May Need Dietary Supplements

As dietitians, we believe in getting nutrients from whole and lightly processed foods. As practical people, we know that can be difficult, especially as you get older and your needs change.

On the whole, Americans don't eat the suggested servings from whole grains, fruits, vegetables, seafood, or dairy on a regular basis. As a result, many women, and men, under-consume calcium, vitamin D, potassium, and dietary fiber.[8] Research also suggests that women lack vitamins A, C, and E, magnesium, and choline.[9, 10]

With time, deficiencies in one or more nutrients may lead to health problems, especially after menopause. According to the Dietary Guidelines for Americans (DGA), dietary supplements and fortified foods, such as breakfast cereals and certain brands of orange juice and eggs, may be useful for providing one or more nutrients missing from your eating plan.[11] You may need one or more dietary supplements if any of the following apply:

- You skimp on a variety of nutrient-rich foods.
- You avoid foods from one or more food groups, such as dairy or grains.
- You limit or avoid all animal products.
- You follow a restricted diet, including a gluten-free eating plan, the Paleo diet, or the ketogenic diet.
- You smoke cigarettes.
- You take certain medications.

MULTIVITAMINS

Multivitamins are the most popular dietary supplement with American adults. "Multivitamins" is actually a misnomer, because these supplements typically contain a mixture of vitamins *and* minerals. Some brands include botanicals, which are plant-based compounds, as well as other ingredients, such as soy isoflavones, which we discussed in chapter 6.[12]

We are fans of multivitamins because they can plug micronutrient gaps, but supplements are no match for a balanced plant-based eating plan. While multivitamins supply a variety of nutrients, they typically come up short on calcium, potassium, choline, and omega-3 fats, and may not contain enough vitamin D. Multivitamins also lack protein, fiber, phytonutrients, and other compounds found in food.

SINGLE-NUTRIENT DIETARY SUPPLEMENTS

A daily multivitamin can cover a lot of bases, but it doesn't always fill in all the blanks. Here are some single nutrient supplements that you may need.

Vitamin D. Many women don't get the vitamin D they require from foods such as milk, salmon, and tuna. Vitamin D helps the body to absorb and use calcium, and with time, even slight shortfalls in vitamin D can put bones at risk for fracture. Vitamin D also supports immunity, cell function, and the nervous system. The body makes vitamin D when skin is exposed to strong ultraviolet B (UVB) rays from the sun. However, it's difficult for many women to produce adequate amounts of vitamin D for reasons we discuss in chapter 7.

Salmon, tuna, and fortified milk supply vitamin D, but you may not eat enough of these foods on a regular basis to meet suggested vitamin D intakes. For example, it takes six 8-ounce glasses of milk to satisfy an adult's daily requirement for vitamin D. It's more reasonable to meet vitamin D needs with a combination of food and supplements. Multivitamins typically contain at least 10 micrograms (400 International Units, or IU) of vitamin D. The recommended amount for women is 15 micrograms (600 IU) daily until age 70, and 20 micrograms (800 IU) per day after that. Women who have been diagnosed with low levels of vitamin D in their blood typically need large amounts in prescription form, and they must take lower levels of vitamin D on a daily basis after that to prevent deficiency. See the list of foods with vitamin D in chapter 7.

Omega-3 fats. Omega-3 fats are necessary for proper blood clotting, helping arteries to relax and contract properly, and for reducing inflammation in the body. Docosahexaenoic acid (DHA), an omega-3 found in the greatest concentrations in brain and retina cells, is vital for brain health, while a combination of DHA and eicosapentaenoic acid (EPA) supports heart health. According to the American Heart Association (AHA), omega-3 fats help to keep the heart beating properly and reduce the risk of erratic rhythms that can lead to sudden death from a heart attack or stroke. Omega-3 fats are also useful in decreasing elevated triglycerides in the blood, slowing plaque formation in the arteries, and possibly lowering blood pressure.[13]

Fish and seafood are the best food sources of DHA and EPA. The Dietary Guidelines for Americans (DGA) recommends eating at least 8 ounces of fish weekly to help prevent heart disease, which would provide, on average, 250 milligrams of combined DHA and EPA a day.[14] Research shows we consume only about 90 milligrams per day.[15] Women who avoid or limit fish may benefit from omega-3 supplements with DHA and EPA. Though there are no U.S. Dietary Reference Intakes for EPA and DHA, the World Health Organization (WHO) suggests adults consume 200 to 500 milligrams a day of combined EPA and DHA.[16] The FDA recommends no more than 2,000 milligrams of DHA and EPA daily from dietary supplements, and possibly less if you take certain medications. Some cardiovascular problems may warrant therapy with much higher doses of fish oil but should be done under medical supervision only.[17]

Choline. Choline supports the liver and the muscles, and is part of cell membranes, which protect the inner workings of cells. It's also the raw material for producing a neurotransmitter that allows cells in the nervous system to communicate with each other.

Animal foods, such as eggs, meat, poultry, and seafood, supply the most choline. Women need 425 milligrams of choline daily, but research from the National Health and Nutrition Examination Survey (NHANES) shows that they consume an average of just 278 milligrams.[18] Menopause may change the body's need for choline, as estrogen is involved in choline production. Research suggests that the choline needs of postmenopausal women are higher than during their premenopausal years. Until choline recommendations account for changes in estrogen levels, concentrate on consuming the suggested amount.[19]

Women who avoid or limit animal foods will likely have a hard time meeting the recommended daily intake for choline. Multivitamins contain little, if any, choline. When purchasing choline supplements, look for them as choline bitartrate to get the most choline for your money.

Calcium. If you don't get enough calcium from foods on a daily basis, you may need a dietary supplement. Calcium supplements come in several forms, including those made with calcium carbonate or calcium citrate. Calcium carbonate is widely available and relatively inexpensive. Calcium carbonate is also found in certain over-the-counter antacid products, including Tums and Rolaids, which, in addition to reducing stomach acid, are reliable calcium sources.

Calcium carbonate is absorbed best when taken with food, while calcium citrate can be consumed with or without food. Calcium citrate malate is a form of calcium typically added to beverages and is well absorbed by the body. Generally speaking, calcium from any type of dietary supplement is best absorbed in doses of 500 milligrams or less at a time.

What Are Probiotics?

Probiotics are live microorganisms that are nearly always bacteria. When probiotics are consumed in adequate amounts, they provide a specific, intended health benefit.[20] The most common probiotics are bacteria that belong to the *Lactobacillus* and *Bifidobacterium* groups.[21] Each of these two broad groups includes many types, or strains, of bacteria. Other bacteria are used as probiotics, and so are yeasts such as *Saccharomyces boulardii*.[22]

Products sold as probiotics include foods with live active cultures and dietary supplements. Probiotics such as *Lactobacillus* may help to prevent diarrhea caused by infections or antibiotics, relieve symptoms

(continued)

of hay fever and ulcerative colitis, lower total and LDL ("bad") cholesterol, and reduce swelling from rheumatoid arthritis in women. Probiotics can also modestly lower blood pressure, especially in people with higher blood pressure to start, and may lessen feelings of depression and anxiety.[23, 24]

With all the buzz about probiotics, it's easy to believe that they colonize the gut, but they are unlikely to take up permanent residence there for a variety of reasons. However, probiotics can promote gut health as long as you consume them on a regular basis and your diet is adequate in fiber to help them thrive. It is important to note that the benefits of probiotics are strain-specific. That means it's necessary to consume a probiotic backed by scientific research that shows it is the correct strain for the desired result. Refer to the Clinical Guide to Probiotic Products Available in U.S.A. at www.usprobioticguide.com for strain-specific information. In addition, taking probiotics supplements without eating enough fiber is like buying a goldfish and never feeding it. You must consume fiber to keep your gut healthy.

While researchers have pinpointed the benefits of specific probiotics in helping with certain chronic conditions, it's unclear how probiotic supplements benefit healthy people. Though probiotics are generally safe, the possibility of side effects exist. Consult your doctor or nurse practitioner before taking probiotic supplements. Resist the urge to use probiotics to treat health issues instead of seeing your healthcare provider for treatment.

Dietary Supplement Safety

While the potential benefits of micronutrient supplements likely outweigh the risks in most cases, there are some safety considerations, including risk of toxicity. If you take more than one dietary supplement, you may be getting excessive amounts of individual nutrients. The best way to figure out your need for dietary supplements is to have a registered dietitian/nutritionist (RDN) evaluate your typical eating pattern to see what's missing. A RDN can also assess if you're going overboard on certain nutrients by evaluating the labels of the dietary supplements and fortified foods you consume. It's helpful to bring your supplement bottles or photos of the ingredient list and dose label to the visit.

Keep a list of your dietary supplements and doses with you to share with health-care professionals because dietary supplements may have negative interactions with certain medications or health conditions. Alert your doctor or nurse practitioner if any of the following apply:

- You also take prescription or over-the-counter medication.
- You're being treated for cancer or you have a history of cancer.
- You're going to have surgery, including dental surgery (tell the dentist).
- You smoke or you did smoke cigarettes.

Never substitute dietary supplements, such as those that promise to lower cholesterol levels, for medications that your doctor or nurse practitioner has prescribed.

Your pharmacist is required to provide a Medication Guide

each time you fill a prescription that describes the drug, potential side effects, and how to avoid them. Some side effects may include interactions with certain nutrients or foods. For example, if you take certain statin drugs (atorvastatin, lovastatin, or simvastatin) to reduce blood cholesterol levels, you should not drink large amounts of grapefruit juice.

Several dietary supplements can interact with the blood-thinning medication warfarin (Coumadin) and alter its effectiveness. The FDA advises people taking warfarin to avoid dietary supplements of garlic, ginger, glucosamine, ginseng, ginkgo, omega-3s, and vitamin E because they enhance the effect of the drug and can increase the chance of bleeding. On the other hand, vitamin K in dietary supplements (and foods) can lower the effectiveness of warfarin. If you take warfarin, talk to a RDN about how to eat a balanced diet that works with your medication and not against it.

According to the FDA, proton pump inhibitors (PPI), such as omeprazole (Prilosec) and lansoprazole (Prevacid), used to treat gastroesophageal reflux disease and peptic ulcer disease, can deplete magnesium from the body. If you take a PPI, ask your doctor or nurse practitioner if you should have your magnesium levels checked. The heart medication digoxin also causes magnesium loss.[25]

PPIs may also interfere with natural vitamin B_{12} absorption from food by slowing the release of gastric acid into the stomach. (Synthetic vitamin B_{12} in fortified foods and dietary supplements does not require stomach acid to digest and absorb.) It's a good idea to get your vitamin B_{12} levels checked if you have taken PPIs for at least a year.[26]

The commonly used diabetes drug metformin can also interfere with vitamin B_{12} absorption, so those on this medication long-term should be routinely screened for B_{12} deficiency.[27]

Prednisone and other corticosteroids, used to manage inflammation and other conditions, may deplete calcium from your bones and impair vitamin D metabolism. Using corticosteroids for long periods may increase bone fracture risk. Speak with your doctor or nurse practitioner about taking supplemental calcium and vitamin D to offset the effects of corticosteroids.[28]

What Are Daily Values?

The Supplement Facts Panel on the package must list the percent Daily Value (DV) for each vitamin, mineral, or other active ingredient. The percent DV is an expression of the amount of the nutrient in one serving of that supplement. For example, if the label lists 25% of the DV for calcium, it means that one serving of that supplement provides 25% of the calcium you need in a day.

DVs for adults are based on nutrient needs for a 2,000-calorie diet for healthy people. The Food and Drug Administration has not set DVs for every nutrient, so there could be blank spaces in the Supplement Facts Panel.

The Supplement Facts Panel must also list the amount of each ingredient, which may be a better tool for evaluating how much of a nutrient you're getting. For example, a supplement with 25% of the DV for calcium supplies 325 milligrams of calcium.

Dietary Supplements for Menopausal Symptoms

Dietary supplements are useful for getting the micronutrients and other nutrients you need, but that's not the only reason why women take them. Many turn to botanicals and other compounds in dietary supplements in an effort to relieve hot flashes, manage mood, and prevent poor sleep.

Women are often interested in whether it's possible to control hot flashes using natural remedies as an alternative to hormone replacement therapy. There's a shortage of research in this area and what does exist is often conflicting.

The nutrients of most interest are isoflavones, found in soy. Asian women report fewer hot flashes and other menopausal symptoms, which could be related to their higher intake of the estrogen-like compounds found in soy foods called isoflavones. There are many healthy reasons to eat soy foods, which are excellent sources of plant protein, but studies have not identified any consistent effect of soy on hot flashes. Using concentrated isoflavone supplements to alleviate hot flashes has also been studied with mixed results. Owing to their higher concentration of estrogen-like compounds, it's best to discuss using concentrated isoflavone supplements with your healthcare provider, particularly if you have any estrogen-related health concerns, such as a history of breast cancer or an elevated risk for the condition.

Herbs like black cohash, dong quai, and ginseng have also been studied as natural remedies for hot flashes, as they may have some estrogen-like action. Research is mixed, but as with isoflavones, any supplement or herb that may affect estrogen levels should be discussed with your healthcare provider to explore the risks or interactions with the medications you take.

Botanical supplements are beyond the scope of this book, but we do want to mention that just because a supplement is "natural" that doesn't make it safe. Any dietary supplement may contain ingredients that can interact with food, medications, or other supplements, and may pose concerns for women with chronic conditions.

How to Choose Dietary Supplements

You have a lot of choice when it comes to dietary supplements. Here are some buying strategies.

- **Pick a reputable brand.** We favor well-known brands with favorable ratings from organizations such as ConsumerLab .com. Avoid supplement companies that make grand claims for their products, which happens to be against FDA rules.
- **Check for seals of approval.** Organizations such as the U.S. Pharmacopeia (USP) test dietary supplement quality. Look for supplements with the USP seal of approval on the label. This indicates that the manufacturer of the product followed standards set by the USP in making the supplement. NSF International, an organization that independently analyzes dietary supplements for quality and purity, allows those that meet their tough testing standards to display the NSF seal.
- **Choose a form.** Micronutrient supplements come as pills, liquids, and chewables, including gummies. Expect ingredients such as gelatin, sweeteners, and cornstarch in gummies. Vitamins and minerals are not tasty, and in most cases sugar is used to mask their taste in chewables and liquids. The more sugar, the less nutrition, as sweet liquid and chewable

supplements typically contain fewer nutrients. However, that may not matter, especially if you have very small nutrient gaps in your diet.

- **Assess the nutrient levels.** It would be nice to pick a multivitamin that supplied 100% or less of the Daily Value. Chances are, you don't need large amounts of many of the nutrients in a multivitamin, including vitamins B_6 and B_{12}, so consider taking half the suggested daily dose. Pick a supplement with the majority of vitamin A from beta-carotene rather than retinol. If you smoke or did in the past, avoid supplements with high levels of beta-carotene, as they have been linked to an increased risk of lung cancer.

- **Check the expiration date.** Opt for a product with the longest shelf life to get the most for your money.

- **Scan the label for other ingredients.** Supplements may include botanicals and inactive ingredients used in their production. Check the label if you're sensitive to colors and fillers, such as those that may contain gluten. Added ingredients such as botanicals often add to the cost and provide little benefit.

11

THE MENOPAUSE DIET PLAN

To this point we've focused on the common health concerns affecting women in the peri- and postmenopausal years, and what the evidence says are the best strategies for achieving and maintaining good health and fitness. Now it's time to pull together what you've read into a cohesive, enjoyable, and personalized plant-based eating plan that's rich in protein, fiber, vitamins, minerals, and other beneficial nutrients, while also low in saturated fat, sodium, and added sugar.

The Details of the Menopause Diet Plan

The Menopause Diet Plan (MDP) is based on the Mediterranean-style of eating that's known to support health in the many ways we've discussed throughout this book. It's a satisfying, energizing, and flexible way to eat that's tailored to women's needs before, during, and after menopause. We covered the highlights of the MDP in chapter 1. Here are some additional details:

- **It's easy to customize.** We offer three approaches to plant-based eating, depending on whether your eating routine needs some tweaking; you would benefit from more structure using a "balanced plate" approach; or you'd prefer a calorie-controlled plan to track food portions.
- **It emphasizes protein.** As discussed in chapter 9, research suggests that midlife and menopausal women need more protein than the current recommended amounts. Each meal in the structured meal plans provides about one-third of your daily protein needs, which will help you feel fuller for longer, preserve muscle mass, and support bone health.
- **It curtails carbohydrates.** The MDP is not a low-carbohydrate diet, but it is lower in carbohydrates than the typical American way of eating, and likely lower than what you've been eating prior to menopause! Being mindful of carbohydrate intake during the menopausal years helps to decrease the risk for prediabetes and diabetes because your body's inclination to gain belly fat decreases its ability to process excess carbohydrate.
- **It promotes eating regularly.** Eating enough during the day and limiting excess calories at night can help balance energy levels and mood, and may help you sleep better. Regular food intake also better aligns with our natural circadian rhythms that regulate metabolism, hormones, and many other bodily functions.
- **It encourages variety.** Balanced eating plans that favor plant foods typically result in a greater diversity of benefi-

cial gut bacteria that support good health. Choosing from an array of whole grains, fruits, vegetables, nuts, seeds, and legumes also supplies the vitamins, minerals, fiber, and phytonutrients you need.

- **It's lower in sodium.** The MDP includes whole and lightly processed foods, which helps to keep sodium intake lower than the typical American diet.
- **It includes healthy fats.** Olive oil is the primary source of fat in the MDP diet plans. While we recommend vegetable oils, including canola and olive, we don't rule out butter and healthy tub spreads. However, we do suggest cooking with healthy oils and using the other fats as condiments in small amounts.

No eating plan is perfect. For example, it's often difficult for menopausal women to get enough calcium from food alone, which would require the equivalent of upwards of four servings of dairy foods daily.

In keeping with a plant-based approach, the MDP suggests two servings of dairy foods daily, which could result in a calcium shortfall. Vitamin D is another nutrient in short supply in the MDP and other eating plans. You may need calcium and vitamin D supplements, especially after menopause when calcium needs increase. See chapter 10 for more on dietary supplements.

Let's Talk Numbers

By this point you can tell we're realists. We've been where you are, or where you're headed, and we know it's probably not possible to go through the menopausal years thinking that, with enough hard work, you can prevent your body from changing. Again, maybe you're one of the lucky few, but we doubt it or you probably wouldn't be reading this book!

Is it harder to lose weight when you're older? Maybe, particularly if you've spent a lifetime avoiding healthier eating and exercising, or if you've always been naturally thin and are dealing with belly fat and weight gain for the first time. But let's face it, managing your weight regardless of age is rarely a cakewalk. Our goal is to help you strike a balance between good health and a good quality of life. Even though it's morphed, your body can still be beautiful, strong, and capable of doing all the things that can make the next phase of life fun, liberating, and adventurous!

CALORIES COUNT, BUT NOT COMPLETELY

When weight control is your goal, calories matter. Anyone can lose weight when she drastically reduces calorie intake, but calorie restriction alone is not enough to help most keep the pounds at bay. In our opinion, you're better off focusing on the what, when, and how's of eating for lasting weight-control success. Of course, we can't talk about weight control without mentioning calories because they matter to energy balance.

A calorie is a measure of energy from food and beverages, and the energy expended in physical activity. Calorie requirements vary based on age, sex, body size, genetics, and activity level. The most accurate way to determine metabolic rate (without including calories burned in activity) is indirect calorimetry, which is generally only available in research units and certain medical settings. Easily available methods of estimating calories are just rough estimates for determining your unique metabolic rate. The one that best matches up with indirect calorimetry is the Mifflin St Jeor[1] calculator, which you can access at https://www.acaloriecalculator .com/. Many popular web- and app-based nutrition tools use this equation, and you can get an estimate of your calorie needs by setting up a profile in a free food and activity logging app, which also generates nutrient goals after you answer questions about your sex, size, weight goals, and level of physical activity.

The Dietary Guidelines for Americans (DGA) also provide calorie estimates for *weight maintenance* based on sex, age, and activity level.[2] Keep in mind that the DGA doesn't account for height, weight, and genetics. And be careful about choosing an activity level. We humans have a natural inclination to overestimate how active we are,[3] which often leads to frustration when it comes to weight control.

The USDA chart divides physical activity into three levels to help determine daily calorie needs. Pick a level that honestly describes you:

- *Sedentary*: The bare minimum of physical activity to get through a typical day.
- *Moderately active*: Physical activity that is equivalent to walking 1.5 to 3 miles daily at the rate of 3 to 4 miles per hour (about 15 to 20 minutes per mile) in addition to the light activity you do to get through a typical day.
- *Active*: Walking more than 3 miles daily at a rate of 15 minutes per mile to 20 minutes per mile (3 to 4 miles per hour) or the equivalent in other exercise, in addition to the light activity you do to get through a typical day.

Estimated Daily Calories to Maintain Weight

AGE (YEARS)	SEDENTARY	MODERATELY ACTIVE	ACTIVE
41–45	1,800	2,000	2,200
46–50	1,800	2,000	2,200
51–55	1,600	1,800	2,200
56–60	1,600	1,800	2,200
61–65	1,600	1,800	2,000
66–70	1,600	1,800	2,000
71–75	1,600	1,800	2,000
76 and up	1,600	1,800	2,000

If you want to lose weight, we recommend eating fewer calories (but never less than 1,600 a day) and increasing your physical activity. As you can see from the chart above, the more you move, the more calories you can eat to maintain your weight.

We feel strongly about not over-restricting your calories to lose weight. Temporary change yields temporary results, so it's important to choose a calorie level you can live with for the long term. Exercise is not optional for weight management or good health.

To support the MDP calorie-structured plan, we've provided details for three calorie levels: 1,600, 1,800, and 2,000 calories, starting on page 214. Choose the plan that comes closest to your needs. Given all the unknowns unique to each of us, you may have to tweak food intake over time to get the desired results, but these plans provide a jumping-off point.

Tracking calories can be helpful in estimating the amount of food that influences your weight. Sadly, it's an imperfect science. If we had a dime for every time a client told us she was counting every calorie and she wasn't losing weight, we'd be very rich women. The reason the math doesn't always work out is due in part to the fact that accurately tracking calories requires weighing and measuring everything you eat, including restaurant food, which is next to impossible. In addition, wearable fitness trackers and machines at the gym may overestimate the number of calories burned. Your genetics and circadian rhythms may also influence whether you burn off excess calories or store them as fat.

That's not to say tracking calories and nutrients isn't helpful. Many studies identify journaling as a powerful tool for helping people transition from being "mindless" to "mindful" eaters, but it's just important to take calorie estimates for both food intake and exercise with a grain of salt, viewing them as a guide, not gospel.

Ultimately, you'll need to figure out what works best for you. It is important to realize, however, that after menopause you will likely need fewer calories than before, and may need to eat less, exercise more, or both to manage your weight.

Is Intermittent Fasting for You?

You've probably heard a lot about various forms of fasting, which are generally referred to as "intermittent fasting," or IF. IF is not a fad or a diet. Rather, it limits when you eat, not so much what you eat. It's an eating pattern that seeks to better align food intake with natural circadian rhythms and allows the body to balance periods

(continued)

of eating with periods of fasting[4] (see chapter 2). There are several types of IF, including:

- *Alternate-day plan*: Fasting every other day of the week.
- *The 5:2 plan*: Eat as usual on five days of the week. Limit calories to 25% of your needs (500 calories on a 2,000-calorie eating plan) on two non-consecutive days, such as Monday and Thursday.
- *Time-restricted eating* (TRE): Limit food intake to a 12-hour window, or shorter, every day. For example, you can choose to eat all your food from 10 a.m. to 6 p.m., or during any other time frame that works for you.

Research on the influence of circadian rhythms and weight is evolving, but much of it suggests potential benefits of corralling calorie intake into a narrower period of time. Research shows condensing food intake into fewer hours over the day may help with weight loss,[5, 6] better regulate blood glucose and prevent diabetes,[7] and may even improve cancer survivorship.[8]

Alternate-day and 5:2 fasting are the most widely studied forms of fasting,[9] but as mentioned, we're wary of eating patterns that are likely hard to adhere to in the long term. In our opinion, TRE is the only form of fasting that has any real-life staying power. According to the theory behind TRE, allowing more hours of fasting may promote weight loss, or prevent gradual weight gain, by reducing the time the body is in calorie-storing mode.

Some people may be able to comfortably wrangle

their eating into eight hours a day, while others may need at least a 12-hour window. Regardless of your goal, we'd like to reinforce a few important points about TRE:

- Start eating earlier in the day with a goal of winding down as early in the evening as possible. Ample research exists to support eating breakfast for easier weight control. We've counseled lots of women who skip breakfast, start eating at noon, and keep at it until 10 p.m. or 11 p.m., and we overwhelmingly feel this pattern is linked to weight gain rather than weight loss.
- No matter how you distribute your food over the day, eating far more calories than you need can easily overrun any metabolic advantages that may come when you stop eating earlier.
- TRE should be a general goal to make you more mindful of eating regularly during the daylight hours, not an overly restrictive rule that makes you feel like you failed if you end up eating later than you would like.

The What, When, and How of the Menopause Diet Plan

It's time to dig into the details of eating to stay healthy and help control your weight at midlife. We hope that you're getting the message: A balanced plant-based eating plan is the way to go. As we walk through the MDP, you'll notice that we emphasize healthy eating patterns, nutritious and delicious food choices, and lasting lifestyle behaviors—and not a strict set of food rules. We like to eat as much as anyone, and we would never tell people to completely avoid certain foods. Foods are not "good" or "bad." Those words are loaded with emotion and have the potential to influence how we feel about ourselves when we're eating.

We take the 80/20 approach to healthful eating—aiming to eat in a way that does the body good roughly 80% of the time and allocating space for foods for pure enjoyment. That doesn't mean that fun foods can't also be healthful! We can think of plenty, including all the MDP recipes in chapter 12. It's also fine to start with small changes, even if you begin with a 50/50, or 40/60 ratio of healthful to "fun" foods!

The MDP Plate

As mentioned, the Menopause Diet Plan offers three approaches to healthy eating: Advice on how to adjust a healthful eating plan to account for menopausal changes, a "balanced plate" approach, and a calorie-oriented approach for those who like a little more structure. If research on the state of the average American diet is any indicator, most peri- and menopausal women could use some help adopting a healthier way of eating.

The MDP plate is a tool for healthy eating during the transition to menopause, and afterward. Our visual depiction of a balanced diet helps simplify the science of what to eat and guides you about what to put on your plate at mealtime. Our plate is inspired by several healthy eating icons you may have seen, including MyPlate, the U.S. government's eating icon, and by the top-rated plant-based eating styles: the Mediterranean plan and the DASH diet.

The Menopause Diet Plan is flexible, and it's possible to customize it to a vegan or vegetarian eating plan and to other plant-based traditional diets such as those consumed in Asia, Latin America, and Africa.[10] No matter what your eating style, if you've avoided whole fruits, vegetables, and whole grains, now is the time to get serious about eating a more varied diet. Check out the About the Food Groups section on page 233 for a list of nutritious foods and suggested portion sizes to put on the MDP plate.

The Menopause Diet Plate

Beverages

Choose water, unsweetened tea, or coffee. Include at least two servings of low-fat and fat-free dairy milk or unsweetened soy milk daily.

Protein
Eat more seafood, poultry, eggs, and moderate amounts of fatty red meat and full-fat cheese. Include plant-based proteins, like legumes, soy foods, nuts, seeds, nut and seed butters, and quinoa (which can count as protein or a whole grain), more often.

Healthy Fats
Healthy fats, such as olive and canola oils, may be added to foods. They are also part of foods such as nuts, seeds, avocados, and fish. Read more about fat in chapter 3.

Grains
Include at least three servings of whole grains, like brown rice, wild rice, quinoa, farro, oats, and whole-grain pasta, cereal, crackers, and tortillas, every day. Look for the word "whole" as the first ingredient on food packages.

Protein

Vegetables

Healthy Fats

Grains

Fruits

Vegetables
Choose non-starchy vegetables, such as broccoli, cauliflower, and carrots, more often. Starchy vegetables, like potatoes, sweet potatoes, winter squash, corn, peas, and plantains, can be enjoyed as a grain alternative if you have prediabetes or diabetes.

Fruits
Eat a variety of whole fruits, and limit juices.

BREAKFAST PLATE

Busy women often skimp on breakfast, so we designed a visual to encourage balance and variety in the first meal of the day. The goal is to pair protein- and grain-rich foods and round out the meal with fruits or vegetables, or a mixture. While portion sizes depend on calorie needs, examples of a balanced breakfast include a veggie and cheese omelet with half or the entire whole-grain English muffin and an apple, a slice or two of whole-grain toast with nut butter and a banana, or a bowl of oatmeal prepared with milk instead of water and topped with chopped nuts and berries. The fruit could also be set aside for later and eaten as a midmorning snack.

The Balanced Breakfast Plate

Protein
Include a source of protein, such as milk, eggs, yogurt, cheese, nuts, seeds, nut or seed butter, legumes, or seafood.

Fruits/Vegetables
Include fruits or vegetables, such as a piece of whole fruit, fruit salad, berries in a smoothie or on cereal, or vegetables in an omelet or on avocado toast.

Grains
Whenever possible, opt for whole grains, such as oats and other cereals, breads, tortillas, English muffins, pancakes, quinoa, and muesli. On food labels, look for "whole" in the first ingredient.

It can be tricky to figure out the food group servings in mixed dishes. We've got you covered! The recipes in chapter 12 provide that information to better help you track what is on your plate and in your glass.

EAT MORE VEGETABLES

In our experience, people struggle to include enough vegetables because they don't have the time to prepare them, they aren't interested, or both. We've devised strategies to make it easier to eat the vegetables you need.

- Keep plain frozen vegetables on hand. You prevent food waste by using only what you need.
- Capitalize on convenience and buy pre-cut fresh vegetables.
- Include ½ cup of leafy greens or half an avocado in a smoothie, or make a pumpkin smoothie with canned pureed pumpkin.
- Snack on hummus. (Garbanzo beans are vegetables!)
- Sip on 100% vegetable juice.
- Roast extra vegetables to add to any meal, omelet, or pizza. For example, toss chopped broccoli, cauliflower, and chopped red and green bell peppers in olive oil and roast at 400°F for 15 to 20 minutes.
- While the oven is on, throw in a few whole sweet potatoes to have later for snacks or with a meal.
- Slice an avocado in half, sprinkle with salt if desired, and enjoy as part of a meal or a snack.
- Make salad a meal. (See How to Make a Meal from Salad, page 275.)

A PLUG FOR PROTEIN

Few people seem to have trouble getting enough protein at dinner, but they lag at breakfast, lunch, and snacks. In addition to providing the raw materials to make muscle, protein keeps you fuller for longer and can slow the rise in blood glucose after a meal or snack. No matter what eating style you choose, aim for at least 20 grams of protein at every meal and include protein in snacks, too. Here are tips for meals that make it easier to include protein.

BREAKFAST

1 small container plain Greek yogurt, ½ cup fresh or frozen raspberries, 1 (1-ounce) slice whole-grain toast with 1 tablespoon peanut butter

½ cup oats microwaved with 8 ounces milk, a small banana, and 1 cooked egg

⅔ cup 1% low-fat cottage cheese, ½ cup chopped fruit or berries, and 2 tablespoons chopped walnuts or slivered almonds

Peanut Butter Smoothie (page 257)

LUNCH/DINNER

Tuna sandwich: 3 ounces canned tuna, drained, on 2 (1-ounce) slices whole-grain bread, and 1 cup baby carrots

Salad: 2 cups greens topped with 3 ounces sliced cooked chicken and 1 (1-ounce) slice whole-grain toast

Whole-wheat wrap (1 ounce) with ⅓ cup hummus, ½ cup black beans, ⅓ cup tabbouleh, 2 tablespoons crumbled feta cheese, romaine lettuce, and roasted red peppers

Stir-Fry, Your Way (page 263), made with shrimp

SNACK SMARTS

We are a nation of snackers. Adults in the United States consume hundreds of calories a day between meals. There's nothing wrong with snacking. We believe in obeying your hunger, and planned, nutritious snacks can help prevent mindlessly eating high-calorie foods with little nutrition. You do need to account for snack calories as part of daily calorie needs, of course.

Combine foods with protein and nutritious carbohydrate-rich foods for healthier snacking. Protein-rich foods, such as dairy products, soy foods, and nuts and nut butters, promote eating satisfaction and supply vitamins and minerals. Nutritious plant-based foods—whole grains, beans, fruit, vegetables, nuts, and seeds— provide phytonutrients, filling fiber, and carbohydrates for energy. Here are some of our favorite snacks:

¾ cup dry-roasted soy nuts (edamame)

½ cup whole-grain cereal and ½ cup milk or unsweetened fortified soy beverage

Trail mix: ¼ cup whole-grain cereal, 2 tablespoons each raisins and nuts

Half a tuna fish or turkey sandwich on whole-grain bread and a handful of cherry tomatoes

1 reduced-fat mozzarella cheese stick and 6 whole-grain crackers

1 hard-cooked egg and a 1-ounce whole-grain roll or slice of toast

1 packet plain one-minute oats prepared in the microwave with 8 ounces milk, topped with 2 tablespoons chopped nuts and sweetener of your choice

Small carton of plain Greek yogurt and ½ cup fresh berries

3 cups low-fat microwave popcorn (popcorn is a whole grain!) tossed with ⅓ cup grated Parmesan cheese

1 cup lentil soup topped with ¼ cup shredded cheddar cheese

½ cup low-fat cottage cheese and 6 whole-grain crackers

10 small whole-grain pretzels and 2 tablespoons hummus

2 tablespoons peanut butter and 6 whole-grain crackers or 10 baby carrots

When to Eat: Timing Matters

As we've discussed, it's clear that other factors besides calories are at play in weight control, including our natural circadian rhythms that tend to prefer a more daytime eating pattern.

Eating three full meals a day (with a snack) used to be standard. People also tended to take their lunch breaks, and many grew up in homes where someone—usually mom—had dinner on the table at a reasonable hour (what a luxury!). Compare that to our current environment, where we may or may not eat breakfast or lunch, which finally catches up with us at midafternoon, when we're at high risk for grabbing a vending-machine snack because we're starved, followed by a fistful of something when we get home and a late dinner that's twice the size of our other meals. Some of us may even dive into an after-dinner snack that's either a segue to relaxation or just something our brain is demanding because we neglected our hunger all day! By the time menopause arrives, many women have developed a night-eating pattern that can collide head-on with their circadian rhythms, preventing weight loss and promoting weight gain with age.

What to Eat: The MDP Method

We don't count every calorie, but we do have a general idea of our calorie needs and think you should, too, especially if you can't understand why you're gaining weight or why you can't take it off. Research shows that the average person is a pretty abysmal calorie estimator, even when it comes to guessing the calories in healthy food. Who among us hasn't given ourself a pass on the portion because the pasta was whole wheat?[11]

As registered dietitians, we're often asked for sample meal plans for healthy eating. We think they can be useful. Even when you don't follow them to the letter, you gain an awareness of what a certain number of calories looks like, and that may help you create parameters for better eating. As we discussed, when it comes to how a particular calorie level may affect your weight, there are no guarantees. Our meal plans are meant to be guides to better eating. If you find it stressful to follow a structured meal plan, don't do it. Stick with the balanced plate approach at meals and snacks instead. Here are some facts about the MDP meal plans:

- All the meal plans derive less than 50% of their calories from carbohydrates and are particularly appropriate for diabetes prevention.
- Afternoon snacks contain carbohydrates and protein to help stabilize blood glucose and hunger levels throughout the day. If the time between lunch and dinner is extra-long, consider adding fruit in the late afternoon to avoid feeling over-hungry when you sit down for dinner.
- Given our goal of encouraging you to wrap up your eating earlier, our meal plans don't include an evening snack. If this doesn't work for you right away, limit your nighttime snack

to 100 calories or so, which amounts to a piece of fruit, a reduced-fat cheese stick, or 3 cups of low-fat microwave popcorn. You could also try a cup of calorie-free herbal tea as an evening snack.

- There is a lot of choice on these meal plans and you can adjust them to fit your needs. If cancer prevention is a priority, avoid processed meats (aside from special occasions) and limit red meat (beef, pork, and lamb) to 12 to 18 ounces per week.

- If you think it might be helpful, log your food intake on a nutrition app, even if just for a few days. Many apps also allow you to record physical activity and provide an estimate of calories burned, which can be factored into your daily calorie goal, if you find that motivating.

- Be flexible. Consider these meals plan a guide for better eating, not something to get overly anxious about if you're not nailing your numbers perfectly. Our plans are not a test of your willpower!

- Added sugar and alcohol supply extra calories and are not included in the meal plans. That's not to say you can't have alcohol and added sugar, but we suggest consuming them in limited amounts.

- Find a list of suggested serving sizes starting on page 234.

The 1,600-Calorie Eating Plan

According to the USDA, this calorie level is the estimated amount for sedentary women over the age of 51 who want to maintain their weight. If weight loss is your goal, increase your physical activity, but don't eat fewer than 1,600 calories a day, regardless of age, because that will increase the risk for nutrient deficiencies. See chapter 9 for suggestions about how to move more. Here are the recommended servings for each food group every day:

Vegetables: 2

Fruit: 2

Grains: 4

Dairy: 2

Protein: 8 servings (ounces) per day, total; with a combination of the following **per week**:

> Seafood: 12 ounces
>
> Meat, poultry, eggs, soy: 40 ounces total
>
> Nuts and seeds: 4 ounces total

Oils: 1½ tablespoons oil, such as olive and canola oil, per day, or a tub spread made with olive oil or other healthy fat that has no trans fat and no more than 2 grams of saturated fat per tablespoon

SAMPLE MEAL PLAN 1: 1,600 CALORIES

BREAKFAST

1 (1-ounce) slice whole-grain toast with 1 tablespoon peanut butter

1 large egg, cooked without added fat

1 small banana, orange, apple, or pear

½ cup 1% low-fat milk or unsweetened soy milk

SNACK
½ cup plain fat-free Greek yogurt

1 cup fresh or wild blueberries

LUNCH
Salad: 2 cups dark green leafy vegetables, such as spinach, kale, and romaine lettuce; 1 medium tomato, sliced; ½ cup chopped cucumber; 3 ounces flaked tuna fish or salmon (canned or pouched); 1 tablespoon olive oil, mixed with balsamic or other vinegar, if desired

1 (1-ounce) whole-grain roll

SNACK
3 cups low-fat microwave popcorn tossed with ⅓ cup shredded cheese

DINNER
1 (4-ounce) boneless, skinless chicken breast, grilled or roasted

1 cup chopped broccoli, carrots, or asparagus, roasted with 1 teaspoon olive oil

½ cup cooked whole-wheat pasta with ¼ cup jarred tomato sauce

SAMPLE MEAL PLAN 2:
1,600 CALORIES

BREAKFAST
Berry and Almond Overnight Oats (page 259)

Or: Microwave ½ cup oats with 1 cup 1% low-fat milk or un-sweetened soy milk. Top with ½ cup berries and 2 teaspoons sliced almonds.

SNACK
1-ounce part-skim mozzarella stick

1 clementine or tangerine

LUNCH
Grain bowl: Layer ½ cup cooked farro, quinoa, or other whole grain; 1 medium tomato, chopped; ½ cup cooked broccoli or other vegetable; 3 ounces cooked chicken. Top with 1 table-spoon olive oil, mixed with balsamic or other vinegar if desired, or 1 tablespoon of prepared peanut sauce or other sauce.

SNACK
1 small pear

¼ cup roasted almonds

DINNER
Ground Turkey and Vegetable Stew (page 278)

1 (1-ounce) slice whole-grain bread or roll with 1 teaspoon heart-healthy spread

SAMPLE MEAL PLAN 3:
1,600 CALORIES

BREAKFAST
½ cup whole-grain, ready-to-eat cereal

1 cup 1% low-fat milk or unsweetened soy milk

1 small banana, apple, orange, or pear

1 large egg, cooked without added fat

SNACK
6 small whole-grain crackers

1 ounce hard cheese, such as cheddar

LUNCH
1 serving leftover Ground Turkey and Vegetable Stew (page 278)

1 (1-ounce) slice whole-grain roll with 1 teaspoon heart-healthy spread

SNACK
Small apple

1 tablespoon peanut or almond butter

DINNER
1 (4-ounce) fish fillet, grilled or roasted

1 cup chopped carrots, cauliflower, or green beans, roasted with 1 teaspoon olive oil

½ cup cooked brown rice, farro, or quinoa, with 1 teaspoon olive oil

SAMPLE MEAL PLAN 4:
1,600 CALORIES

BREAKFAST

Peanut Butter Smoothie (page 257)

SNACK

½ cup whole-grain cereal

¾ cup 1% low-fat milk or unsweetened soy milk

LUNCH

Sandwich: 3 ounces lean roast beef or sliced turkey breast on 2 (1-ounce) slices whole-wheat bread, 1 teaspoon mayonnaise, lettuce, tomato, and onion if desired

1 cup baby carrots (about 12)

SNACK

½ cup 1% low-fat milk or unsweetened soy milk

Small apple or pear

¼ cup chopped walnuts

DINNER

Stir-Fry, Your Way (page 263), made with tofu

½ cup cooked brown rice

SAMPLE MEAL PLAN 5:
1,600 CALORIES

BREAKFAST

½ cup oats cooked in the microwave with 1 cup 1% low-fat milk or unsweetened soy milk and topped with ¼ cup raisins and 1 tablespoon chopped walnuts

1 large egg, cooked without added fat

SNACK

2 clementines or tangerines or 1 large orange

LUNCH

1 serving leftover Stir-Fry, Your Way (page 263)

½ cup cooked brown rice

SNACK

6 whole-wheat crackers

1 ounce hard cheese, such as cheddar

DINNER

4 ounces shrimp or sliced boneless, skinless chicken breast, sautéed in 1 tablespoon olive oil and minced fresh garlic, mixed with 1 cup steamed chopped broccoli, served over ½ cup cooked whole-wheat pasta

The 1,800-Calorie Eating Plan

According to the USDA, women ages 51 years and older who are moderately active and those who are 41 to 50 years old who are sedentary may maintain their weight on 1,800 calories daily. Women ages 41 to 50, and 60 and older who are moderately active may lose weight at this level. Here are the recommended servings for each food group each day:

Vegetables: 2½

Fruit: 2

Grains: 4

Dairy: 2

Protein: 9 servings (ounces) per day, total; with a combination of the following **per week**:

> Seafood: 15 ounces
>
> Meat, poultry, eggs, soy: 44 ounces total
>
> Nuts and seeds: 4 ounces total

Oils: 2 tablespoons oil, such as olive and canola oil, per day, or a tub spread made with olive oil or other healthy fat that has no trans fat and no more than 2 grams of saturated fat per tablespoon

SAMPLE MEAL PLAN 1:
1,800 CALORIES

BREAKFAST
1 (1-ounce) slice whole-grain toast with 1 tablespoon peanut butter

1 large egg, cooked without added fat

1 small banana, apple, orange, or pear

½ cup 1% low-fat milk or unsweetened soy milk

SNACK
½ cup plain fat-free Greek yogurt

1 cup fresh or wild blueberries

LUNCH
Salad: 2 cups dark green leafy vegetables, such as spinach, kale, and romaine lettuce; 1 medium tomato, sliced; ½ cup chopped cucumber; ¼ cup garbanzo beans; 3 ounces flaked tuna fish or salmon (canned or pouched); 1 tablespoon olive oil mixed with balsamic or wine vinegar if desired

1 (1-ounce) whole-grain roll with 1 teaspoon heart-healthy spread

SNACK
3 cups low-fat microwave popcorn tossed with ⅓ cup grated Parmesan cheese

DINNER

1 (5-ounce) boneless, skinless chicken breast, grilled or roasted

1½ cups chopped broccoli, carrots, or asparagus, roasted with 2 teaspoons olive oil

½ cup cooked whole-wheat pasta with ¼ cup jarred tomato sauce

SAMPLE MEAL PLAN 2: 1,800 CALORIES

BREAKFAST

Berry and Almond Overnight Oats (page 259)

Or: Microwave ½ cup oats with 1 cup 1% low-fat milk or unsweetened soy milk. Top with ½ cup berries and 2 teaspoons sliced almonds.

SNACK

1-ounce part-skim mozzarella stick

2 clementines or tangerines or 1 large orange

LUNCH

Grain bowl: Layer ½ cup cooked farro, quinoa, or other whole grain; 1 medium tomato, chopped; 1 cup cooked chopped broccoli or other vegetable; and 4 ounces cooked chicken. Top with 4 teaspoons olive oil, mixed with balsamic or other vinegar if desired, or 1 tablespoon of prepared peanut sauce or other sauce.

SNACK

1 small pear

¼ cup roasted almonds

DINNER

Ground Turkey and Vegetable Stew (page 278)

1 (1-ounce) slice whole-grain bread or roll with 1 teaspoon heart-healthy spread

SAMPLE MEAL PLAN 3: 1,800 CALORIES

BREAKFAST

½ cup whole-grain, ready-to-eat cereal

1 cup 1% low-fat milk or unsweetened soy milk

1 small banana, apple, orange, or pear

1 large egg, cooked without added fat

SNACK

6 small whole-grain crackers

1 ounce hard cheese, such as cheddar

LUNCH

1 serving leftover Ground Turkey and Vegetable Stew (page 278)

1 (1-ounce) whole-grain roll with 1 teaspoon heart-healthy spread

SNACK

Small apple or pear

2 tablespoons peanut or almond butter

DINNER

1 (5-ounce) fish fillet, grilled or roasted

1½ cups chopped carrots, cauliflower, or green beans, roasted with 2 teaspoons olive oil

½ cup cooked brown rice, farro, or quinoa, with 1 teaspoon olive oil

SAMPLE MEAL PLAN 4: 1,800 CALORIES

BREAKFAST

Peanut Butter Smoothie (page 257)

SNACK

½ cup whole-grain ready-to-eat cereal

1 cup 1% low-fat milk or unsweetened soy milk

½ cup berries

LUNCH

Sandwich: 3 ounces lean roast beef or sliced turkey breast, 2 (1-ounce) slices whole-grain bread, 2 teaspoons mayonnaise, lettuce, tomato, and onion if desired

1 cup baby carrots (about 12)

SNACK

1 cup 1% low-fat milk or unsweetened soy milk

Small apple or pear

¼ cup chopped walnuts

DINNER

Stir-Fry, Your Way (page 263), made with tofu

½ cup cooked brown rice

SAMPLE MEAL PLAN 5:
1,800 CALORIES

BREAKFAST

½ cup oats cooked in the microwave with 1 cup 1% low-fat milk or unsweetened soy milk and topped with ¼ cup raisins and 2 tablespoons chopped walnuts

1 large egg, cooked without added fat

SNACK

2 clementines or tangerines or 1 large orange

LUNCH

1 serving leftover Stir-Fry, Your Way (page 263)

½ cup cooked brown rice

SNACK

6 whole-wheat crackers

1½ ounces hard cheese, such as cheddar

DINNER

5 ounces shrimp or sliced boneless, skinless chicken breast, sautéed in 4 teaspoons olive oil and diced garlic and mixed with 1 cup steamed chopped broccoli, served over ½ cup cooked whole-wheat pasta

What Works for Us

I was mortified when I gained 10 pounds after menopause. I ate healthy foods and exercised five days a week, but menopause had other ideas for my body. I took an honest look at my diet and made some changes. I started following a version of the 1,800-calorie MDP, which increased my fiber consumption and nearly doubled my protein intake; even today, it helps prevent mindless nibbling that contributes to excess calories. I still eat chocolate every day, but about half as much as I did, and I don't feel deprived at all!

—Liz

The 2,000-Calorie Eating Plan

According to the USDA, women ages 41 to 50 years who are moderately active and those who are 61 years and older but very active may maintain their weight on this plan. Here are the recommended servings for each food group each day:

Vegetables: 2½

Fruit: 2½

Grains: 5

Dairy: 2

Protein: 10 servings (ounces) per day, total; with a combination of the following **per week**:

> Seafood: 15 ounces
>
> Meat, poultry, eggs, soy: 50 ounces total
>
> Nuts and seeds: 5 ounces total

Oils: 2½ tablespoons oil, such as olive and canola oil, per day, or a tub spread made with olive oil or other healthy fat that has no trans fat and no more than 2 grams of saturated fat per tablespoon

SAMPLE MEAL PLAN 1: 2,000 CALORIES

BREAKFAST

2 (1-ounce) slices whole-wheat toast with 2 tablespoons peanut butter

1 large egg, cooked without added fat

1 small banana, apple, orange, or pear

½ cup 1% low-fat milk or unsweetened soy milk

SNACK

½ cup plain fat-free Greek yogurt

1 cup fresh or wild blueberries

LUNCH

Salad: 2 cups dark green leafy vegetables, such as spinach, kale, and romaine lettuce; 1 medium tomato, sliced; ½ cup chopped cucumber; ¼ cup garbanzo beans; 4 ounces flaked tuna fish or salmon (canned or pouched); 4 teaspoons olive oil mixed with balsamic or other vinegar if desired

1 (1-ounce) whole-grain roll with 1 teaspoon heart-healthy tub spread

SNACK

3 cups low-fat microwave popcorn tossed with ⅓ cup grated Parmesan cheese

Small apple

DINNER

1 (6-ounce) boneless, skinless chicken breast, grilled or roasted

2 cups chopped broccoli, cauliflower, or asparagus, roasted with 1 tablespoon olive oil

1 cup cooked whole-wheat pasta with ¼ cup jarred tomato sauce

SAMPLE MEAL PLAN 2:
2,000 CALORIES

BREAKFAST

Berry and Almond Overnight Oats (page 259)

Or: Microwave ½ cup oats with 1 cup 1% low-fat milk or unsweetened soy milk; top with ½ cup berries and 2 teaspoons sliced almonds.

SNACK

1-ounce part-skim mozzarella stick

2 clementines or tangerines or 1 large orange

LUNCH

Grain bowl: Layer 1 cup cooked farro, quinoa, or other whole grain; 1 medium tomato, chopped; 1 cup cooked chopped broccoli or other vegetable; and 4 ounces cooked chicken. Top with 4 teaspoons olive oil mixed with balsamic or other vinegar if desired, or 1 tablespoon of prepared peanut sauce or other sauce.

SNACK

1 small pear

¼ cup roasted almonds

DINNER

Ground Turkey and Vegetable Stew (page 278)

1 (1-ounce) slice whole-grain bread or roll with 2 teaspoons heart-healthy spread

SAMPLE MEAL PLAN 3: 2,000 CALORIES

BREAKFAST

½ cup whole-grain, ready-to-eat cereal

1 cup 1% low-fat milk or unsweetened soy milk

1 small banana, apple, orange, or pear

1 large egg, cooked without added fat

SNACK

6 small whole-grain crackers

1 ounce hard cheese, such as cheddar

LUNCH

1 serving leftover Ground Turkey and Vegetable Stew (page 278)

1 (1-ounce) whole-grain roll with 1 teaspoon heart-healthy spread

SNACK

Small apple or pear, sliced, dipped in 2 tablespoons peanut or almond butter and rolled in 2 tablespoons raisins

DINNER

1 (5-ounce) fish fillet, grilled or roasted

2 cups chopped carrots, cauliflower, or green beans, roasted with 2 teaspoons olive oil

1 cup cooked brown rice, farro, or quinoa, with 1 teaspoon olive oil

SAMPLE MEAL PLAN 4: 2,000 CALORIES

BREAKFAST

Peanut Butter Smoothie (page 257)

SNACK

½ cup whole-grain ready-to-eat cereal

1 cup 1% low-fat milk or unsweetened soy milk

1 cup berries

LUNCH

Sandwich: 3 ounces lean roast beef or sliced turkey breast, 2 (1-ounce) slices whole-wheat bread, 1 (1-ounce) slice cheese, 2 teaspoons mayonnaise, lettuce, tomato, and onion if desired

1 cup baby carrots (about 12) and 2 tablespoons hummus for dipping

SNACK

1 cup 1% low-fat milk or unsweetened soy milk

Medium apple or pear

¼ cup chopped walnuts

DINNER

Stir-Fry, Your Way (page 263), made with tofu

1 cup cooked brown rice

SAMPLE MEAL PLAN 5: 2,000 CALORIES

BREAKFAST

½ cup oats cooked in the microwave with 1 cup 1% low-fat milk or unsweetened soy milk and topped with ¼ cup raisins and 3 tablespoons chopped walnuts

1 large egg, cooked without added fat

SNACK

2 clementines or tangerines or 1 large orange

LUNCH

1 serving leftover Stir-Fry, Your Way (page 263)

½ cup cooked brown rice

SNACK

6 whole-wheat crackers

1½ ounces hard cheese, such as cheddar

DINNER

5 ounces shrimp or sliced boneless, skinless chicken breast, sautéed in 4 teaspoons olive oil and diced fresh garlic, mixed with 1½ cups steamed chopped broccoli, served over 1 cup cooked whole-wheat pasta

About the Food Groups

The following information about foods and their portions sizes from the USDA will help you easily tailor a plan to suit your eating style. For those who may be familiar with the American Diabetes Association (ADA) Exchange Lists for meal planning, the portion sizes for carbohydrate-containing foods are similar for most foods. Where discrepancies exist, differences are identified with an asterisk in the food group lists. For example, USDA considers 1 cup of juice as a serving, whereas ADA serving sizes are ½ cup or less, depending on the juice.

GRAINS

Grains provide carbohydrates, the body's preferred energy source, and contain a variety of nutrients, including fiber, phytonutrients, and B vitamins. Grains from cookies, cake, and pastry are considered treats, as they contain added sugars and fats while offering little healthful nutrition. See the following list for grain foods and their portion sizes, which are equal to 1 serving.

FOOD TYPE	SERVING SIZE
Bagel	1 ounce (e.g., 1 mini bagel or ½ a 2-ounce bagel)*
Biscuits	1 small (2 inches in diameter)
Bread	1 regular slice or 1 small slice French or 4 snack-size slices
Cornbread	1 small piece (2½ x 1¼ × 1¼ inches)
Crackers	5 whole-wheat crackers or 2 rye crisp breads or 7 square or round crackers
English muffin	½ muffin
Grains, such as rice, bulgur, quinoa, teff, barley, freekeh	½ cup cooked
Oatmeal (regular or quick-cooking)	½ cup cooked or 1 instant packet or 1 ounce (⅓ cup) dry
Pancakes	1 medium (4½-inch diameter) or 2 small (3-inch diameter)
Pasta (includes couscous)	½ cup cooked or 1 ounce dry
Popcorn	3 cups popped

Ready-to-eat cereal	1 cup flakes or rounds or 1¼ cups puffed
Rice	½ cup cooked or 1 ounce dry
Tortillas	1 small (6-inch)

*Keep in mind that the average 3½- to 4-inch deli bagel weighs 3 to 4 ounces, equal to 3 to 4 servings.

Are Refined Grains Okay to Eat?

While the MDP encourages whole-grain intake, it is possible to incorporate your favorite refined grains, like white pasta, rice, and bread, in a healthy plant-based eating plan. A 2019 study found that when considered on their own as opposed to part of an unhealthy eating plan, there is no evidence to link refined grains with type 2 diabetes, cardiovascular disease, stroke, or high blood pressure.[12]

However, like the members of other food groups, refined grains are not all created equal. It's important to distinguish between refined grains that are staples of a balanced eating plan, such as bread, cereal, and pasta, and refined grains that we dietitians consider indulgences, such as cookies, cake, and other sweets. Indulgences are packed with added sugar and fat and tend

(continued)

to offer little nutrition for the calories, while everyday staples are fortified with vitamins and minerals, and are significant sources of several B vitamins and iron.

No single food can ruin a healthy eating plan, and overall eating patterns matter most to health. Experts recommend consuming six servings of grains daily on a 2,000-calorie pattern and making half of the grains you eat whole grains no matter what your calorie intake.[13] That means there's room for refined grains in a balanced diet, including occasional indulgences. Enjoy!

VEGETABLES

Vegetables supply fiber, potassium, vitamin C, magnesium, and phytonutrients, among other nutrients. It's important to eat a variety of vegetables. For example, green leafy vegetables are rich in vitamin K to support bone health. Legumes, such as garbanzo beans, soybeans, and black beans, are rich in fiber and also supply protein. Paler produce, such as mushrooms, onions, and cauliflower, provide an array of nutrients, too. Most vegetables are very low in carbohydrate and are considered "free" for those curbing their carbohydrate intake to help prevent or manage diabetes. If you need to control your blood glucose levels, you should consider that the following starchy vegetables are higher in carbohydrate content: potatoes, sweet potatoes/yam, winter squash, corn, peas, and plantains.

FOOD TYPE	SERVING SIZE
Broccoli	1 cup chopped or florets, *or* 3 (5-inch) spears, raw or cooked
Kale, collard greens, mustard greens, turnip greens	1 cup cooked
Raw leafy greens: spinach, romaine, watercress, dark green leafy lettuce, endive, escarole	2 cups raw *or* 1 cup cooked
Carrots	2 cups raw *or* 1 cup cooked; 1 cup raw or cooked strips, slices, or chopped; *or* 2 whole medium; *or* 1 cup baby carrots (about 12)
Pumpkin	1 cup cooked and mashed
Red peppers	1 cup chopped, raw or cooked, *or* 1 large pepper
Tomatoes	1 large whole, *or* 1 cup chopped or sliced raw, canned, or cooked
Tomato juice	1 cup
Sweet potato	1 large baked, *or* 1 cup cooked, sliced, or mashed
Winter squash (acorn, butternut, Hubbard)	1 cup cooked
Beans, dried, and peas (black beans, garbanzo, kidney, pinto, soybeans, black-eyed, split, lentils)	1 cup cooked, whole or mashed

FOOD TYPE	SERVING SIZE
Corn, yellow or white	1 cup *or* 1 large ear
Green peas	1 cup
Potatoes	1 cup cooked diced or mashed, *or* 1 medium, boiled or baked*
Cabbage, green	1 cup raw or cooked, chopped or shredded
Cauliflower	1 cup florets, raw or cooked
Celery	1 cup raw or cooked, diced or sliced, *or* 2 large stalks
Cucumbers	1 cup raw, sliced, or chopped
Green or wax beans	1 cup cooked
Green peppers	1 cup chopped, raw, or cooked, *or* 1 large pepper
Lettuce, iceberg	2 cups shredded or chopped
Mushrooms	1 cup raw or cooked
Onions	1 cup raw or cooked
Summer squash or zucchini	1 cup cooked

*The ADA considers a serving of potato to be ½ cup cooked, diced or mashed, or ½ of a medium potato.

FRUIT

Fruit contains carbohydrates, fiber, potassium, vitamins A and C, and phytonutrients. All forms of fruit, including fresh, frozen, canned, dried, and juiced, are good for you, although it's best to limit juice to a serving or less per day in favor of plain, whole fruits. Many fruits, such as bananas, apples, and pears, require little preparation and are portable. Choose fruits without added sugar, such as unsweetened applesauce and canned fruits packed in 100% fruit juice, and raisins.

FOOD TYPE	SERVING SIZE
Apple	½ large (3¼ inches), *or* 1 small (2½ inches), *or* 1 cup sliced, raw or cooked
Applesauce*	1 cup
Banana*	1 large (8 to 9 inches), *or* 1 cup sliced
Berries (excluding strawberries)	1 cup
Cantaloupe	1 cup diced or balls
Grapes	1 cup whole or cut up, *or* 32 seedless grapes
Grapefruit*	1 medium, *or* 1 cup sections
Orange	1 large, *or* 1 cup sections
Orange, mandarin	1 cup, drained canned
Peach	1 large (2¾ inches), *or* 1 cup raw, cooked, or drained canned; *or* 2 halves, canned
Pear	1 medium; *or* 1 cup raw, cooked, or drained canned, sliced or diced
Pineapple	1 cup raw, cooked, or drained canned, chunks, sliced, or crushed
Plum	1 cup sliced raw or cooked; *or* 3 medium; *or* 2 large

FOOD TYPE	SERVING SIZE
Strawberries	8 large *or* 1 cup fresh or frozen, whole, halved, or sliced
Watermelon	1 small wedge (1 inch); *or* 1 cup diced or balls
Dried fruit	¼ cup
100% fruit juice*	1 cup

*The ADA considers a serving of 100% fruit juice to be ⅓ to ½ cup, depending on the type; a serving of applesauce is ½ cup unsweetened; a banana is 1 small; and a grapefruit serving is ½ of a whole fruit.

DAIRY

You might be surprised to find soy "milk" in the dairy group. While they are dairy-free, soy beverages with added calcium, vitamin A, and vitamin D are included because their nutritional profiles are similar to dairy milk. The members of the dairy group also supply protein and potassium. Vitamin D is added to nearly all dairy milk and many plant milks, and to some brands of yogurt, but it's not added to cheese. Sour cream and cream cheese aren't included in the dairy group because they don't contain enough calcium to qualify. See the following list for servings in the dairy group. Choose lower-fat dairy foods to limit saturated fat intake.

SERVING SIZE

1 cup milk

½ cup evaporated milk

1 cup (8 ounces) yogurt*

1½ ounces hard cheese, such as cheddar, mozzarella, Swiss, or Parmesan

1 cup calcium-fortified soy milk

⅓ cup shredded cheese

2 ounces processed cheese (e.g., American)

½ cup ricotta cheese

2 cups cottage cheese

*Single-serve yogurt containers are often 6 ounces or less, which counts as just ¾ cup of dairy. Greek yogurt has nearly twice the protein and less calcium than regular yogurt.

Are Plant Milks Good for You?

Chances are, the only milk you drank growing up came from a cow. Now, there's an array of plant "milks" to choose from, and it's important to understand how they differ from dairy milk, and what they have to offer.

Plant milks are produced by grinding beans, grains, or nuts, and blending them with water and other additives, such as sugar, vitamins, and minerals. With the exception of soy milk, the biggest difference between most types of plant milk and dairy milk concerns protein. For example, 1 cup of almond milk, coconut milk, or rice milk has about 1 gram of protein, while a cup of dairy milk supplies 8 grams. Oat milk has about 2 grams of protein. While protein levels vary, calcium and vitamin D levels in fortified plant milk are often quite similar to dairy milk.

Generally speaking, unsweetened soy milk with added calcium and vitamin D is the closest to dairy milk. Check the Nutrition Facts label and ingredient list for added sugars and other additives in plant-based milks, which are more costly than dairy milk.

PROTEIN

Protein is found in animal and plant foods, including meat, poultry, seafood, legumes, eggs, soy products, nuts, and seeds. Plant-based eating capitalizes on the diversity of foods found in the protein group.

While it's not essential to avoid meat and poultry, it is important to include adequate amounts of plant protein and fish. Each meal plan in the MDP explains how much seafood to eat weekly, as well as how much meat, poultry, eggs, soy foods, and nuts and seeds.

Protein is also found in dairy foods. If you avoid dairy and you don't drink soy milk, you may not be consuming the level of protein we consider adequate for menopausal and perimenopausal women. Add 2 ounces of protein foods to your daily eating plan and take calcium and vitamin D supplements to help make up for what you're missing by avoiding dairy products. (See chapter 10 for more on dietary supplements.)

FOOD TYPE	SERVING SIZE EQUAL TO 1 OUNCE OF PROTEIN
Lean cooked beef or pork	1 ounce
Cooked chicken or turkey, without skin	1 ounce
Sliced turkey sandwich meat	1 ounce
Cooked fish or shellfish	1 ounce
Eggs*	1 whole
Nuts	½ ounce (12 almonds, 24 pistachios, or 7 walnut halves)

Seeds (pumpkin, sunflower, or squash)	½ ounce
Peanut butter or almond butter	1 tablespoon
Beans and peas (black beans, kidney beans, white beans, etc., or garbanzo beans, lentils, or split peas, etc.)	¼ cup cooked
Baked beans, refried beans	¼ cup
Tofu	½ cup (about 2 ounces)
Tempeh	1 ounce cooked
Roasted soybeans	½ cup
Falafel patty	1 (2¼ inches, 4 ounces)
Hummus	2 tablespoons

*Three large egg *whites* equal 2 ounces of protein. We suggest eating yolks to get all the vitamins, minerals, choline, lutein, and zeaxanthin that eggs provide.

FATS AND OILS

Fats and oils are not a food group, but they do provide essential nutrients and make food satisfying and tasty. Some foods, such as nuts, olives, fish, and avocados, supply healthy fats.

Solid fats are hard at room temperature. Most solid fats, such as butter, are made from animal foods and tend to have more saturated fat than healthier oils. Saturated plant fats, like coconut and palm oil, should be limited.

Healthy tub spreads are okay as condiments, but it is preferable to use healthy oils such as olive oil and canola oil for cooking. Oils, even the healthy kind, as well as other sources of added fat, are high in calories, so use them mindfully.

Helpful Strategies for Implementing the Menopause Diet Plan

We've discussed in detail how diet and physical activity choices can influence your health for better or worse, and we have offered a variety of ways to transition to a healthier lifestyle. But knowing and doing are two different things. Behavior change can be a bumpy and stressful road. To help you navigate the MDP in a determined but forgiving manner, we offer the following strategies. We hope they resonate with you.

STRATEGY 1: RESPECT YOUR HUNGER

It's critical to view hunger as a cue to eat, not something to be ignored. Tending to hunger sooner rather than later may help you eat more slowly and notice when you're starting to feel full. To determine how often you should eat, rate your hunger on a scale of 1 to 10 (1 = "not hungry" and 10 = "starving"). The goal is to eat your next meal or snack when your hunger is a 5 or 6 ("somewhat hungry"), instead of waiting for the 8 to 10 "starved" hunger that often leads to overeating, which often happens at night and isn't in line with circadian rhythms.

For some people, eating every four hours or so helps keep hunger in check. For others, it might be every three or five hours. The idea is to eat as often as needed to keep from feeling starved, and then eating more calories than you need.

STRATEGY 2: ADJUST YOUR ATTITUDE TO AVOID "I'M A FAILURE" SYNDROME

According to National Weight Control Registry (NWCR) founder Dr. Rena Wing, successful weight-losers are encouraged to view lapses as opportunities to learn, not evidence of weakness. We can't emphasize enough the importance of this. People who lose weight and keep it off tend not to view lapses as personal failures but, rather, chances to reflect on what has happened and why, whether it was avoidable, and what they might do differently next time!

STRATEGY 3: FAIL TO PLAN, PLAN TO FAIL!

Relying too heavily on willpower to help you eat healthfully is an approach generally doomed to fail because humans did not evolve to resist food. Your good intentions to choose nutritious foods are commendable, but they will be flattened when you speed through your day, not thinking about food until you're desperately hungry.

Planning is the foundation of a healthy lifestyle, as it proactively sets us up with food options throughout the day. Establish one behavior at a time, and think of the eating outcome you're aiming for as the last domino in a row to fall. Identify what each domino before that last one should look like. For example, to avoid grabbing lunch on the fly, you need to plan time to shop, then prepare and pack the food to bring with you. All this takes time!

STRATEGY 4: KEEP A JOURNAL

Many studies have identified food journaling as helpful for keeping healthy eating on the radar. Journaling can be as simple as toting around a colorful notebook or using an app.

Similar to workplace audits, tracking your food and beverage intake is like conducting an audit of your habits through the day. Writing it all down helps you figure out what's working well and what needs to change.

How to Pair the MDP with Your Online Logging Platform

Popular online nutrition logging platforms include My Fitness Pal, Lose It, Good Measures, Weight Watchers Online, My Net Diary, Apple Watch, My Food Diary, Sparkpeople, and Fitbit's food tracking app. Most have web- or smartphone app-based options. Nutrition apps set nutrient goals, generally based on height, weight, sex, and weight goals, and provide feedback on how you're doing. To find the right fit, experiment. If you don't like the flow of the app, you won't use it. Apps may also provide helpful reminders to eat, drink, or log; pop-up nutrition tips; set up reminders of your goals; or offer ways to network with other users.

STRATEGY 5: TO PRIORITIZE HEALTH, SOMETHING'S GOT TO GIVE

Most of us lead super-busy lives, making meal planning and exercise seem like just more demands on our time. While we can always find time to watch TV or surf the Internet, we need to determine our priorities to practice self-care. The time to purchase and prepare food, exercise, and sleep—even relax—should be budgeted into your day like all the other things you feel are important.

STRATEGY 6: NEVER GIVE UP!

According to Tufts University nutrition researcher Dr. Margo Woods, sticking with significant dietary change is a result of traveling through a three-step process.[14] The process begins with purging highly processed foods from your diet and is followed by adding healthier choices, thereby improving one meal or snack at a time. You will eventually arrive at phase three: consistently eating healthier. Unfortunately, most people get through the first two phases and don't make it to being consistent (which can include occasionally eating whatever you want just because it tastes good!). We know it can be hard to stick with a healthier eating plan when you don't get quick results, but hang in there. It takes time to figure out what will work for you long term.

STRATEGY 7: MANAGE YOUR MIND-SET AND EXPECTATIONS

Making diet and lifestyle changes can be difficult, especially if you have years of failed "diets" under your belt. It can be hard to shake off negative thinking and overly ambitious expectations. But you can't change the past, only learn from it. Focus on getting through one day at a time rather than a long-term goal that you don't even know is doable yet.

Take a positive approach by focusing more on adding nutritious foods to your diet rather than taking tasty foods away. Accept that the process takes time. If you add enough foods that are nutritious and filling, eventually there will be less room for the less desirable stuff.

What Works for Us

Rather than focusing too much on the scale, I try to pay attention to what my body is telling me. Having more energy, sleeping better, and not feeling bloated from overeating after meals are big quality of life boosters for me.

—Hillary

STRATEGY 8: TRUST THAT YOU'RE THE EXPERT IN YOU AND THE GOAL IS NOT PERFECTION

Start building your plan by taking stock of your past experiences, including those things you found helpful (maybe shopping more consistently, exercising in the morning, not buying foods you'd like to limit) and discarding the things that didn't (crash dieting, diet shakes, excessive exercise). Be realistic: You know what behaviors have a chance of lasting and which ones don't.

STRATEGY 9: DON'T GO IT ALONE

Having a helpful spouse, partner, family member, friend, group, therapist, or exercise buddy can be an invaluable asset. Personal coaching provided by a registered dietitian/nutritionist (RDN) can be tremendously helpful. (Trust us, we know!) You can find a RDN in your area on the Academy of Nutrition and Dietetics website, at www.eatright.org, Find an Expert link.

How to Dine Out with Health in Mind

We love to go out to eat, so we're aware of how hard it can be to eat restaurant or take-out food and control your weight, fat, sodium, and added sugar intake.

You know that fast-food joints and chain restaurants are nutritional landmines, but sit-down establishments are, too. A 2016 analysis of meals on the menu at 123 non-chain restaurants in three large American cities found the average meal served up about 1,200 calories, and that didn't include drinks, appetizers, and dessert![15] The biggest offenders? Meals at American, Chinese, and Italian places (our favorites!) averaged about 1,500 calories, or nearly an entire day's worth of calories for most menopausal women!

Regardless of where you eat, remember these two very important points:

1. Portions are probably 30 to 50% larger than you need.
2. The amount of fat, salt, and added sugar is likely a lot higher than experts suggest.

That said, it is possible to dine out and still eat healthfully. All it takes is planning, determination, and these tips to avoid doing dietary damage to your eating plan:

- **Do your homework.** Identify restaurants with lighter, healthier fare, especially if you dine out on a regular basis.

Chain restaurants are mandated by law to provide nutrition information for menu items. Unfortunately, restaurants with fewer than twenty locations aren't.

- **Don't go in ravenous.** When you're really hungry, your power to avoid large amounts of tasty food will be sorely challenged. Eat a light snack that pairs carbohydrates with protein, such as a small apple and peanut butter, or baby carrots and hummus, an hour or so before you go out.
- **Decide on a drink limit** (we're thinking one, or none!) and stick to it. Who needs to drink their calories?
- **Wait until the meal arrives for a cocktail or glass of wine.** Drinking on an empty stomach may lead you to throw caution to the wind when ordering. (Been there!)
- **When you're with a crowd, order first.** It reduces the temptation to order what everyone else is having.
- **Start with soup.** Broth-based soups, such as chicken noodle or egg drop soup, are low in calories and make a great pre-meal filler. Avoid calorie-dense creamed soups, bisques, and chowders.
- **If you don't know how something is prepared, by all means, ask.** Don't be afraid to request that an entrée be prepared with less fat or salt or to make substitutions to lower the carbohydrate or calorie content of a meal.
- **Choose alternatively.** Order a salad and split an entrée. Choose lighter-fare items, or an appetizer, such as shrimp cocktail, and a large garden salad.
- **Take some of it home.** To reduce the temptation to eat more than you should, ask the server to pack up half of a large entrée in a take-home container *before* he brings the food to the table.
- **Order a kid's meal.** At fast-food joints, order a kid's meal

(with fruit, not fries, and plain milk), which is often enough food for many women!

- **Avoid all-you-can-eat buffets.** Why tempt yourself?
- **Choose wisely.** Look for entrées that are steamed, broiled, baked, grilled, braised, roasted, or poached, and avoid those described as stuffed, pan-fried, fried, crispy, crunchy, or sautéed.
- **Avoid fattening side dishes.** Watch for and avoid these terms: fried, scalloped, au gratin, in a cream or cheese sauce, twice-baked, casserole, and tempura-style.
- **Pump up the vegetables.** Take the balanced-plate approach: Ask to double up on the veggies, such as broccoli or carrots, and forgo the bread or pasta.
- **Order whole grains.** Choose brown or wild rice, quinoa, whole-wheat tortillas, and whole-wheat pasta whenever possible.
- **Focus on fat.** It's easy to go overboard with butter, olive oil, and sour cream. Every tablespoon of butter or olive oil adds about 125 calories, and 2 tablespoons of sour cream contributes 50. Ask for dressing on the side, and dip your fork into it before grabbing a bite of salad. You will use less. Ask for sauces on the side, too.
- **Watch the carbs.** If you can't resist the bread, limit yourself to one piece, or roll, and order non-starchy vegetables in place of rice, potato, or pasta to limit carbohydrates. Avoid fatty breads like croissants and gooey rolls and pastries.
- **Go for smart salads.** Salads can have just as many calories and just as much fat as some entrees! They can be smart choices, as long as you limit or avoid fatty pasta and potato salads, croutons, bacon bits, and dressings.
- **Divvy up dessert.** We are suckers for sweets, but we're never

really that hungry after a restaurant meal. If you can't resist, share dessert with as many people as possible. Sometimes, just a bite suffices!

Looking for healthy meal options? Check out healthydining finder.com, a website that compiles dietitian-approved restaurant foods from all over the country and offers the nutrition breakdown for each. Another resource that we love for every kind of cuisine imaginable is *Eat Out, Eat Well,* a book by our fellow dietitian Hope Warshaw.

That's a Wrap!

Whew! We know this chapter, and this book, is packed with information. It may seem like a lot to tackle, but we believe working toward healthier habits during the transition to menopause and afterward is an investment in your future.

We don't get to choose to avoid menopause and aging, but we can choose how we take care of our bodies to add quality to our years. Of course, there are no guarantees in life, but healthy living is an odds game with loads of proven benefits, and that's a gamble we hope you take!

12

THE MDP RECIPES
AND EATING TIPS

D o you have about 30 minutes (and possibly less!) on most days to devote to preparing delicious and nutritious foods that will help you control your weight, stabilize your hormones, and feel better? We think you're probably shaking your head yes, and that's good, because it doesn't take much more than a half hour to make the majority of our recipes that are perfect for midlife, menopausal women and their families.

Our collection is plant-based, but it's not free of animal foods. We're all about flexibility, which is why we've designed recipes that you can prepare several ways. The same goes for salt and added sugar. We keep both to a minimum in our cooking, but you can adjust them to suit your tastes. For the most part, we cook only with heart-healthy oils and encourage you to do the same.

It's not always easy to determine how a serving of food made from a recipe translates to a serving when you're using a balanced-plate approach to meal planning. We have provided that information at the end of each recipe in this chapter with the exception of fat. Fats and oils are added to food and they are also part of foods, including nuts and oils. We also share notes about healthful ingredients, preparation tips, and serving suggestions. No time to cook? We've got you covered with how to assemble nutritious meals and snacks.

We hope that you love these recipes as much as we do, and that you alter them to fit your needs!

BREAKFAST

Dr. Wright's Best Orange-Cranberry Nut Muffins

Makes 12 muffins

Hillary's dad considers making muffins very early in the morning as one of his retirement hobbies. These muffins are a good source of fiber and are delicious with eggs!

1 cup all-purpose flour

¾ cup whole-wheat flour

¼ cup unprocessed bran

½ cup sugar, plus 1 teaspoon for topping (optional)

1 teaspoon baking soda

1½ teaspoons baking powder

½ teaspoon salt

1 cup dried cranberries

½ cup chopped walnuts

1 cup buttermilk

⅓ cup vegetable oil, such
as canola

1 large egg

Zest of 1 orange

1 teaspoon orange extract

1 teaspoon vanilla extract

¼ teaspoon ground
cinnamon (optional)

1. Preheat the oven to 375°F. Line a 12-cup standard muffin tin with paper liners.
2. In a large bowl, combine the flours, bran, ½ cup sugar, baking soda, baking powder, salt, cranberries, and walnuts.
3. In a medium bowl, combine the buttermilk, oil, egg, orange zest, orange extract, and vanilla.
4. Add the buttermilk mixture to the flour mixture and stir until just combined. Do not overmix. Distribute the batter evenly among the muffin cups. If desired, mix 1 teaspoon sugar and the cinnamon in a small bowl, then sprinkle a bit of it on top of each muffin.
5. Bake for 16 to 18 minutes, or until a toothpick inserted in the middle of a muffin comes out clean. Place on a wire rack to cool for 15 minutes before eating.

PER MUFFIN:

Calories: 221

Carbohydrate: 35 grams

Dietary fiber: 3 grams

Total fat: 9 grams

Saturated fat: 1 gram

Cholesterol: 16 milligrams

Protein: 4 grams

Sodium: 283 milligrams

Calcium: 55 milligrams

Added sugar: 8 grams

**INCLUDES THE FOLLOWING SERVINGS
FROM THE FOOD GROUPS:**

Grains: 2 servings

Protein: ½ serving

Wild Blueberry–Banana Oatmeal Bars

Makes 12 bars

The MIND diet calls out berries, including wild blueberries, as particularly protective of the brain. We love wild blueberries because they're delicious and available year-round in the frozen-food aisle! Serve these with a dollop of Greek yogurt.

3 cups quick or old-fashioned rolled oats

½ teaspoon salt

2 teaspoons baking powder

½ teaspoon ground cinnamon (optional)

3 ripe medium bananas, mashed well

¼ cup canola oil

2 large eggs

1 teaspoon vanilla extract

2 cups 1% low-fat milk

3 cups frozen wild blueberries or fresh blueberries

1. Preheat the oven to 350°F. Coat a 9 by 11-inch baking pan with cooking spray.
2. In a large bowl, combine the oats, salt, baking powder, and cinnamon, if using. Set aside. In a separate large bowl, whisk the mashed bananas, oil, eggs, and vanilla until well combined. Whisk in the milk.
3. Pour the banana mixture into the oat mixture. Stir well to combine. Gently add the blueberries. The batter will be soupy. Transfer the batter to the baking pan.
4. Bake for 25 to 30 minutes, or until set. Remove from the oven and place on a wire rack for 15 minutes to cool. Cut into 12 equal-size pieces. (To enjoy later, place in an airtight container and store in the refrigerator.)

PER BAR:

Calories: 194

Carbohydrate: 28 grams

Dietary fiber: 4 grams

Total fat: 7 grams

Saturated fat: 1 gram

Cholesterol: 33 milligrams

Protein: 5 grams

Sodium: 210 milligrams

Calcium: 118 milligrams

Added sugar: 0 grams

INCLUDES THE FOLLOWING SERVINGS FROM THE FOOD GROUPS:

Fruit: ½ serving

Grains: ½ serving

Protein: about 1 serving

Peanut Butter Smoothie

Serves 1

This frothy drink features peanut butter, which helps support heart health. Pair this satisfying sipper with a slice of whole-grain toast for a meal.

½ cup plain fat-free Greek yogurt

¼ cup 1% low-fat milk

2 tablespoons natural peanut butter (without added sugar, if desired)

1 frozen medium banana

½ teaspoon vanilla extract

Place all the ingredients in a blender or food processor and blend on high speed for 45 seconds or until smooth.

PER SERVING:

Calories: 394

Carbohydrate: 42 grams

Dietary fiber: 5 grams

Total fat: 18 grams

Saturated fat: 4 grams   Sodium: 78 milligrams
Cholesterol: 53 milligrams   Calcium: 348 milligrams
Protein: 23 grams   Added sugar: 0 grams

**INCLUDES THE FOLLOWING SERVINGS
FROM THE FOOD GROUPS:**
Dairy: 1 serving   Protein: about 3 servings
Fruit: 1 serving

Tips for Sensational Smoothies

We think the most nutritious smoothies combine foods rich in protein and calcium with fruits and vegetables. This is especially true if you rely on smoothies as a meal or as a substantial part of one. We recommend dairy products, such as milk and yogurt, or fortified unsweetened soy beverages as a base. Plant-based beverages, such as almond or oat milk, are lower in protein and other nutrients, too.

Here's a simple way to assemble a better-for-you beverage. In a blender or food processor, blend 1 cup fresh or frozen (frozen makes for a frothier drink) unsweetened fruit or plain vegetables, such as spinach or kale, or a combination, and mix with ½ cup milk or unsweetened fortified soy beverage and ½ cup plain fat-free Greek yogurt. Add half a scoop of whey protein powder, or other protein powder, for additional protein. Once you've mastered the basics, try adding uncooked oats, nuts, tahini, or unsweetened cocoa powder.

Berry and Almond Overnight Oats

Serves 1

Oats are a humble food with mighty abilities, including lowering blood cholesterol and the risk for heart disease. With crunchy sliced almonds and delectable berries, these overnight oats are a welcome sight when you've got no time in the morning to make breakfast!

½ cup quick or old-fashioned rolled oats

½ cup 1% low-fat milk

¼ cup plain fat-free Greek yogurt

Sweetener of choice, as desired

½ cup fresh raspberries, sliced strawberries, blackberries, or blueberries, or a combination

2 teaspoons sliced almonds

Combine the oats, milk, yogurt, and sweetener in a container with a lid, such as a mason jar. Shake or stir until well combined. Refrigerate overnight. Add the fruit and almonds just before eating.

PER SERVING:

Calories: 299

Carbohydrate: 44 grams

Dietary fiber: 9 grams

Total fat: 7 grams

Saturated fat: 2 grams

Cholesterol: 9 grams

Protein: 17 grams

Sodium: 79 milligrams

Calcium: 268 milligrams

Added sugar: 0 grams

INCLUDES THE FOLLOWING SERVINGS
FROM THE FOOD GROUPS:

Dairy: 1 serving

Fruit: ½ serving

Grains: 2 servings

Protein: about 2½ servings

Cheese and Vegetable Egg Cups

Serves 6

Eggs are rich in protein and choline. One of these egg cups contains nearly as much calcium as a glass of milk and is low in carbohydrates.

¾ cup low-fat cottage cheese

2 teaspoons olive oil

1 medium onion, chopped

20 cherry tomatoes, cut in half

3 large eggs

1 (9-ounce) package frozen chopped spinach, defrosted and well drained

1 cup shredded reduced-fat mozzarella cheese or other hard cheese

½ teaspoon freshly ground black pepper

1. Preheat the oven to 400°F. Coat 6 jumbo muffin cups with cooking spray.
2. Place the cottage cheese in a blender or food processor. Blend for about 45 seconds, or until smooth.
3. In a small skillet, heat the oil over medium heat. Add the onion and tomatoes. Sauté for 5 minutes.
4. In a large bowl, whisk the eggs until just beaten. Add the cottage cheese, onion and tomato mixture, the spinach, cheese, and pepper. Mix well.
5. Divide the egg mixture evenly among the 6 muffin cups. Bake about 20 minutes, or until firm. Remove from the oven and place on a wire cooling rack for 5 minutes. Remove the egg cups from the pan and cool for 5 more minutes.
6. Eat right away or store, covered, in the refrigerator. Reheat for 3 minutes in the microwave, if desired.

PER SERVING:

Calories: 151

Carbohydrate: 7 grams

Dietary fiber: 2 grams

Total fat: 9 grams

Saturated fat: 4 grams

Cholesterol: 108 milligrams

Protein: 13 grams

Sodium: 288 milligrams

Calcium: 230 milligrams

Added sugar: 0 grams

**INCLUDES THE FOLLOWING SERVINGS
FROM THE FOOD GROUPS:**

Dairy: 1 serving

Protein: 2 servings

Avocado Toast, Two Ways

Serves 1

We love avocado toast even more when there's protein involved.

¼ cup low-fat cottage cheese, or 1 egg, fried over easy or scrambled

1 (1-ounce) slice whole-grain bread, toasted

½ ripe avocado, pitted and sliced

Salt and freshly ground black pepper (optional)

1. Place the cottage cheese in a blender or food processor and blend until smooth, about 45 seconds.
2. Spread the cottage cheese on the toast. Top with the avocado and salt and pepper, if desired. As an alternative, top the toast with the avocado and the cooked egg.

PREPARED WITH COTTAGE CHEESE AND AVOCADO:

Calories: 131

Cholesterol: 2 milligrams

Carbohydrate: 17 grams

Protein: 12 grams

Dietary fiber: 2 grams

Sodium: 393 milligrams

Total fat: 2 grams

Calcium: 92 milligrams

Saturated fat: 1 gram

Added sugar: 0 grams

INCLUDES THE FOLLOWING SERVINGS FROM THE FOOD GROUPS:

Grains: 1 serving

Protein: about 1½ servings

Vegetable: ½ serving

PREPARED WITH EGG AND AVOCADO:

Calories: 168

Cholesterol: 187 milligrams

Carbohydrate: 16 grams

Protein: 11 grams

Dietary fiber: 2 grams

Sodium: 226 milligrams

Total fat: 7 grams

Calcium: 83 milligrams

Saturated fat: 2 grams

Added sugar: 0 grams

INCLUDES THE FOLLOWING SERVINGS FROM THE FOOD GROUPS:

Grains: 1 serving

Protein: about 1½ servings

Vegetable: ½ serving

LUNCH AND DINNER

Stir-Fry, Your Way

Serves 4

You can make this recipe four ways, including with tofu. Soy foods pack potassium, magnesium, and phytoestrogens, which act like a weaker form of the estrogen your body produces. Look for tofu processed with calcium for a significant amount of the bone-building mineral. A recent study confirms that eating 25 grams of soy protein daily reduces LDL ("bad") cholesterol, which helps reduce the risk for heart disease.[1]

¼ cup 100% orange juice

3 tablespoons reduced-sodium soy sauce

3 tablespoons rice vinegar

4 large garlic cloves, minced

2 teaspoons peeled, minced fresh ginger

¼ cup cornstarch

2 tablespoons canola oil

1 pound shelled and deveined raw shrimp; or 1 pound boneless top round steak, trimmed of fat and sliced into ¼ by 1-inch pieces; or 1 pound boneless, skinless chicken breast, cut into ½-inch cubes; or 1 (14-ounce) package extra-firm tofu, drained and cut into 1-inch cubes

5 cups chopped vegetables (such as red, green, and orange bell peppers; sugar snap peas; broccoli florets; sliced carrots)

1. In a small mixing bowl, combine the orange juice, soy sauce, vinegar, garlic, ginger, and cornstarch.
2. Heat 1 tablespoon of the oil in a large skillet over medium-high heat. Add the shrimp, steak, or chicken, and cook until the shrimp is opaque, steak is medium rare, or chicken is cooked through, about 5 minutes. (Don't add tofu until the very end.) Transfer the shrimp, steak, or chicken to a plate and cover to keep warm.
3. Add the remaining tablespoon oil to the skillet. Add the vegetables and sauté over medium-high heat for 3 to 4 minutes, or until they are crisp-tender.
4. Add the orange juice mixture to the pan and continue to cook the vegetables until they are fork-tender, stirring constantly, another 3 to 4 minutes. Stir the shrimp, steak, or chicken into the pan and toss with the vegetables to heat through for about 1 more minute. If using tofu instead, add it now, tossing to combine, cover, and cook for 2 minutes, or until heated through.

PER SERVING (WITH SHRIMP):

Calories: 286	Cholesterol: 214 milligrams
Carbohydrate: 24 grams	Protein: 31 grams
Dietary fiber: 4 grams	Sodium: 595 milligrams
Total fat: 8 grams	Calcium: 124 milligrams
Saturated fat: 1 gram	Added sugar: 0 grams

INCLUDES THE FOLLOWING SERVINGS FROM THE FOOD GROUPS:
Protein: about 4 servings
Vegetables: 1 serving

PER SERVING (WITH BEEF):

Calories: 356	Dietary fiber: 4 grams
Carbohydrate: 24 grams	Total fat: 13 grams

Saturated fat: 3 grams

Cholesterol: 87 milligrams

Protein: 38 grams

Sodium: 545 milligrams

Calcium: 63 milligrams

Added sugar: 0 grams

INCLUDES THE FOLLOWING SERVINGS FROM THE FOOD GROUPS:

Protein: about 5½ servings

Vegetables: 1 serving

PER SERVING (WITH CHICKEN):

Calories: 321

Carbohydrate: 24 grams

Dietary fiber: 4 grams

Total fat: 9 grams

Saturated fat: 1 gram

Cholesterol: 87 milligrams

Protein: 36 grams

Sodium: 570 milligrams

Calcium: 45 milligrams

Added sugar: 0 grams

INCLUDES THE FOLLOWING SERVINGS FROM THE FOOD GROUPS:

Protein: about 5 servings

Vegetables: 1 serving

PER SERVING (WITH TOFU):

Calories: 284

Carbohydrate: 26 grams

Dietary fiber: 5 grams

Total fat: 14 grams

Saturated fat: 2 grams

Cholesterol: 0 milligrams

Protein: 17 grams

Sodium: 475 milligrams

Calcium: 417 milligrams

Added sugar: 0 grams

INCLUDES THE FOLLOWING SERVINGS FROM THE FOOD GROUPS:

Protein: about 2½ servings

Vegetables: 1 serving

Beef and Mushroom Chili

Serves 6

Did you know that mushrooms are one of the few natural food sources of vitamin D? They stand in for some of the meat in this fiber-filled chili.

8 ounces 95% lean ground beef or 100% ground turkey breast

½ teaspoon salt

½ teaspoon freshly ground black pepper

1 tablespoon canola or olive oil

8 ounces baby bella mushroom caps, washed and minced

1 large onion, chopped

4 garlic cloves, minced

½ teaspoon ground cumin

½ teaspoon dried oregano

1 large red bell pepper, cored, seeded, and chopped into 1-inch pieces

1 large yellow bell pepper, cored, seeded, and chopped into 1-inch pieces

1 (15-ounce) can black beans, drained and rinsed

1 (15-ounce) can red kidney beans, drained and rinsed

1 (28-ounce) can no-salt-added diced tomatoes

1. Place a large skillet over medium-high heat. Add the meat, breaking it up into very small pieces, and cook for 7 to 10 minutes, or until completely browned. Season with salt and pepper, and stir to combine. Remove the meat from the pan and set aside.

2. Add the oil to the skillet. Add the mushrooms and sauté until they are fork-tender, about 10 minutes. Add the onion and sauté for 2 minutes, until translucent. Add the garlic, cumin,

and oregano, and cook, stirring constantly, for another minute until garlic is soft. Add the bell peppers and continue to cook until they are soft, about 2 minutes more.

3. Add the beans, tomatoes, and meat to the pan. Stir to combine thoroughly. Cover and simmer over low heat for about 20 minutes, stirring occasionally, until the chili is bubbling and aromatic.

PER SERVING (WITH BEEF):

Calories: 336	Cholesterol: 33 milligrams
Carbohydrate: 46 grams	Protein: 25 grams
Dietary fiber: 14 grams	Sodium: 675 milligrams
Total fat: 6 grams	Calcium: 122 milligrams
Saturated fat: 2 grams	Added sugar: 0 grams

INCLUDES THE FOLLOWING SERVINGS FROM THE FOOD GROUPS:

Protein: about 3½ servings
Vegetables: 1½ servings

PER SERVING (WITH TURKEY):

Calories: 325	Cholesterol: 27 milligrams
Carbohydrate: 46 grams	Protein: 26 grams
Dietary fiber: 14 grams	Sodium: 676 milligrams
Total fat: 5 grams	Calcium: 122 milligrams
Saturated fat: 1 gram	Added sugar: 0 grams

INCLUDES THE FOLLOWING SERVINGS FROM THE FOOD GROUPS:

Protein: about 3½ servings
Vegetables: 1½ servings

Salmon and Vegetable Sheet Pan Dinner

Serves 4

A delicious dinner with only one pan to wash? Sign us up! This quick and simple preparation is strong on omega-3 fats and provides more than 40% of the vitamin D you need in a day.

2 tablespoons reduced-sodium soy sauce

3 tablespoons canola oil

1 tablespoon honey or maple syrup

1 tablespoon lime juice (juice of 1 small lime)

4 garlic cloves, minced

1 teaspoon grated fresh ginger

¼ teaspoon paprika

1 (1-pound) salmon fillet, skin on

1 teaspoon toasted sesame oil

4 cups chopped broccoli florets

5 cups peeled and chopped sweet potato, in 1-inch pieces

Salt and freshly ground black pepper

1. Preheat the oven to 400°F. Line a large rimmed baking sheet with parchment paper and coat with cooking spray.
2. In a medium bowl, combine the soy sauce, 1 tablespoon of the canola oil, the honey, lime juice, garlic, ginger, and paprika. Place the salmon in the bowl and coat the skinless side with the marinade.
3. In a large bowl, combine the remaining 2 tablespoons canola oil, the sesame oil, broccoli, and sweet potato. Season to taste with salt and pepper. Toss to coat the vegetables with the oil mixture.
4. Spread the vegetables on the baking sheet in a single layer. Roast for 12 minutes. Create a space in the middle of the sheet

for the fish and place the fillet skin side down. Drizzle any leftover marinade over the salmon and vegetables. Return the baking sheet to the oven to roast for an additional 15 minutes, or until the salmon is opaque in the center and flakes slightly. Serve at once.

PER SERVING:

Calories: 620

Carbohydrate: 78 grams

Dietary fiber: 13 grams

Total fat: 20 grams

Saturated fat: 2 grams

Cholesterol: 70 milligrams

Protein: 34 grams

Sodium: 556 milligrams

Calcium: 161 milligrams

Added sugar: 4 grams

INCLUDES THE FOLLOWING SERVINGS FROM THE FOOD GROUPS:

Protein: about 5 servings

Vegetables: 2 servings

Spaghetti Carbonara with Vegetables

Serves 2

Olive oil is the main fat source in both the Mediterranean style of eating and our MDP. In addition to being a healthy fat, olive oil packs polyphenols—compounds that act as antioxidants, which defend the cells from damage.

4 ounces whole-wheat spaghetti or other pasta

2 tablespoons olive oil

4 garlic cloves, minced

1 yellow bell pepper, cored, seeded, and chopped into ½-inch pieces

2 cups cherry tomatoes, cut in half

4 large eggs

½ cup grated Parmesan cheese

Pinch of red pepper flakes (optional)

¼ cup fresh basil leaves, chopped

1. Cook the pasta according to package directions.
2. While pasta is cooking, heat the oil in a large skillet over medium heat. Add the garlic, bell pepper, and tomatoes, and cook, stirring frequently, until soft, 5 to 7 minutes.
3. Place the eggs in a small bowl and whisk until lightly beaten.
4. When the pasta is ready, drain and transfer it to the skillet using tongs. Toss with the vegetable mixture. Slowly whisk in the eggs while tossing the spaghetti mixture. Cook for another 1 to 2 minutes, until the eggs appear scrambled.
5. Remove the pan from the heat. Sprinkle on the Parmesan cheese, red pepper flakes (if using), and the basil. Serve immediately.

PER SERVING:

Calories: 551

Carbohydrate: 58 grams

Dietary fiber: 7 grams

Total fat: 27 grams

Saturated fat: 8 grams

Cholesterol: 208 milligrams

Protein: 24 grams

Sodium: 522 milligrams

Calcium: 271 milligrams

Added sugar: 0 grams

INCLUDES THE FOLLOWING SERVINGS FROM THE FOOD GROUPS:

Grains: 2 servings

Protein: about 3½ servings

Vegetables: 2 servings

Easy Baked Fish

Serves 4

Here's a super-simple fish dish that's ready in less than 30 minutes. It pairs perfectly with a quick-cooking grain, like quinoa, and a large salad.

1 (1-pound) fillet cod, haddock, or other white fish, skin removed if present

¼ cup plain bread crumbs

¼ teaspoon salt

1 (14.5-ounce) can no-salt-added diced fire-roasted tomatoes

2 tablespoons olive oil

1 tablespoon dried parsley, or 2 tablespoons fresh

1. Preheat the oven to 400°F. Line a medium baking dish with a sheet of foil big enough to overlap the edges and make a packet, such as 12 to 14 inches long by about 8 inches wide.
2. Place the fish fillet in the baking dish.
3. In a small dish, combine the bread crumbs and salt. Sprinkle it evenly over the fish in the pan. Top with the tomatoes, olive oil, and a sprinkling of the parsley.
4. Fold the sides of the foil over the fish, then fold the top and bottom to cover the fish completely. Pinch the foil closed to seal the packet.
5. Bake for 18 to 20 minutes; carefully open the packet slightly to test that the fish is flaky and opaque. Remove from the oven and open the packet carefully to avoid the steam or spilling the juices. Cut into 4 sections and serve immediately.

PER SERVING:

Calories: 214

Carbohydrate: 11 grams

Dietary fiber: 1 gram

Total fat: 8 grams

Saturated fat: 1 gram

Cholesterol: 55 milligrams

Protein: 24 grams

Sodium: 286 milligrams

Calcium: 29 milligrams

Added sugar: 0 grams

INCLUDES THE FOLLOWING SERVINGS FROM THE FOOD GROUPS:

Protein: about 3½ servings

Vegetables: ½ serving

Grilled Chicken with Walnut Pesto Sauce

Serves 4

Walnuts are associated with a lower risk for depression,[2] a healthier gut,[3] and a reduced risk for heart disease,[4] not to mention they are also delicious! Adding yogurt to the pesto keeps the calories reasonably low without sacrificing flavor.

1 cup fresh basil leaves

½ cup roughly chopped walnuts

1 garlic clove

¼ teaspoon salt

2 tablespoons fresh lemon juice

¼ cup grated Parmesan cheese

2 tablespoons olive oil

½ cup plain fat-free Greek yogurt

Pinch of red pepper flakes

1 pound boneless, skinless chicken breast, grilled

1. Place the basil, walnuts, garlic, salt, lemon juice, cheese, and oil in a food processor and blend on high speed until smooth, about 1 minute. Add the yogurt and red pepper flakes, and blend for another 15 to 20 seconds. Refrigerate until ready to use.

2. When ready to serve, top warm grilled chicken with the walnut pesto sauce.

PER SERVING:

Calories: 348

Carbohydrate: 4 grams

Dietary fiber: 1 gram

Total fat: 21 grams

Saturated fat: 4 grams

Cholesterol: 109 milligrams

Protein: 37 grams

Sodium: 323 milligrams

Calcium: 106 milligrams

Added sugar: 0 grams

INCLUDES THE FOLLOWING SERVINGS FROM THE FOOD GROUPS:

Protein: about 5 servings

Chicken Italiano

Serves 6

This is a super-easy, all-in-one skillet recipe that's loaded with vegetables and protein. Serve with whole-wheat pasta or additional vegetables. The dinner will please the whole family and is even better the next day as leftovers!

1½ pounds boneless, skinless chicken breast, cut into 1½-inch cubes

⅓ cup reduced-fat Italian salad dressing

3 tablespoons olive oil

2 garlic cloves, minced

1 medium onion, chopped

2 cups sliced button mushrooms

2 cups sliced zucchini

1 (14.5-ounce) can no-salt-added seasoned diced tomatoes

½ cup reduced-sodium chicken broth

1 tablespoon Italian seasoning

¼ teaspoon salt

⅛ teaspoon freshly ground black pepper

1 cup grated part-skim mozzarella cheese

1. In a medium bowl, combine the chicken with the salad dressing. Place in the refrigerator to marinate for 15 minutes.
2. In a large skillet, heat 2 tablespoons of the oil over medium heat. Add the garlic and onion, and sauté until tender, about 3 minutes. Add the chicken and continue to sauté for 5 to 7 minutes, or until lightly browned. Remove the chicken mixture from the pan.
3. Add the remaining tablespoon oil to the skillet over medium heat. Add the mushrooms and zucchini, and sauté until tender. Return the chicken and toss with the mushrooms and zucchini. Add the tomatoes, broth, Italian seasoning, salt, and pepper and combine well.
4. Turn the heat to low and sprinkle the mixture with the cheese. Cover the pan with a lid or foil and simmer for 6 to 8 minutes, or until the chicken is cooked through and the cheese is melted. Serve.

PER SERVING:

Calories: 365

Carbohydrate: 9 grams

Dietary fiber: 2 grams

Total fat: 17 grams

Saturated fat: 5 grams

Cholesterol: 109 milligrams

Protein: 42 grams

Sodium: 489 milligrams

Calcium: 176 milligrams

Added sugar: 0 grams

**INCLUDES THE FOLLOWING SERVINGS
FROM THE FOOD GROUPS:**

Protein: 6 servings

Vegetables: ½ serving

How to Make a Meal from Salad

We see it all the time: Women lunching on a bowl of light green lettuce topped with a few cucumbers, tomatoes, olives, and croutons, a smattering of cheese, and some salty salad dressing. A few hours later, they're at the vending machine or the drive-through for more food because they are starving! Salad is fine as a side dish, but if you sometimes rely on it for a meal, here are some suggestions for getting more nutrition at the same time and for feeling satisfied longer.

- Use at least 2 cups of dark green leafy vegetables, including kale, spinach, and romaine, green leaf, red leaf, or Boston lettuce.

(continued)

- Add at least ½ cup of diced green, red, orange, or yellow bell peppers, diced tomatoes, sliced carrots, beets, broccoli, or cauliflower, or any combination.
- Layer on some chopped fresh fruit, such as apples or pears, fresh berries, or drained canned fruit, including mandarin oranges and pineapple chunks.
- Top with at least 3 ounces of a protein-rich food, including cooked chicken, canned or pouched tuna or salmon, or tofu.
- Use a small amount of cheese, nuts, or dried fruit as a garnish, if desired.
- Top with a drizzle of 2 teaspoons of olive oil and as much vinegar as you like, or use reduced-fat salad dressing.
- Pair the salad with a small whole-grain roll and a glass of dairy milk, fortified unsweetened soy milk, or a cup of yogurt.

Now, that's a meal!

Lazy Lentil Soup

Serves 4

Lentils double as both vegetable and protein source, and using the canned type gets this soup on the table in about 20 minutes. (Hint: Make a double batch and freeze the rest.) Pair this hearty soup with yogurt and fruit for a complete meal.

2 tablespoons olive or canola oil

1 medium yellow onion, chopped

2 garlic cloves, minced

2 large carrots, cut into ¼-inch pieces

½ teaspoon dried thyme

1 cup cooked lentils, canned or fresh

1 (15-ounce) can no-salt-added diced fire-roasted tomatoes

1½ cups reduced-sodium chicken or vegetable broth

2 packed cups baby spinach

½ teaspoon salt

Freshly ground black pepper

1. In a large skillet, heat the oil over medium-high heat. Add the onion, garlic, and carrots, and sauté for about 5 minutes. Add the thyme and continue to cook until the carrots are fork-tender, another 5 to 7 minutes.

2. Add the lentils, tomatoes, and broth, cover, and cook for about 10 minutes over medium heat. Add the spinach, salt, and pepper. Stir until the spinach is wilted, then serve.

PER SERVING:

Calories: 171

Carbohydrate: 21 grams

Dietary fiber: 6 grams

Total fat: 7 grams

Saturated fat: 1 gram

Cholesterol: 0 milligrams

Protein: 7 grams

Sodium: 373 milligrams

Calcium: 78 milligrams

Added sugar: 0 grams

INCLUDES THE FOLLOWING SERVINGS FROM THE FOOD GROUPS:

Protein: 1 serving

Vegetables: ½ serving

Ground Turkey and Vegetable Stew

Serves 4

This filling recipe checks the boxes for protein, fiber, and vegetables, and it's delicious! There's a reason it's the first dish Hillary taught her three sons how to cook! Serve with a green salad and whole-grain bread.

3 tablespoons olive oil

3 garlic cloves, minced

1 large onion, chopped

1 cup chopped celery

2 cups sliced carrots

2 cups sliced zucchini

1 pound ground 100% turkey breast

1 (28-ounce) can seasoned no-salt-added diced tomatoes

3 cups reduced-sodium beef broth

¼ cup tomato paste

¼ teaspoon salt

½ teaspoon freshly ground black pepper

1½ tablespoons Italian seasoning

1 (15-ounce) can kidney beans, drained and rinsed

1. In a Dutch oven, heat 2 tablespoons of the oil over medium-high heat. Add the garlic and sauté until lightly browned, about 3 minutes. Add the onion and celery, and sauté until tender, another 3 minutes. Add the carrots and zucchini, and continue to cook until slightly tender, about 5 minutes more. Remove the vegetables from the pan.
2. Heat the remaining tablespoon oil in the Dutch oven. Add the turkey, breaking up the meat into very small pieces, and cook until no longer pink, about 5 minutes.

3. Add the vegetable mixture to the Dutch oven along with the tomatoes, broth, tomato paste, salt, pepper, and Italian seasoning. Turn the heat to low, cover, and simmer for 10 minutes, or until the vegetables are crisp-tender. Add the beans and simmer for another 20 minutes, or until heated though.

PER SERVING:

Calories: 420

Carbohydrate: 38 grams

Dietary fiber: 9 grams

Total fat: 13 grams

Saturated fat: 2 grams

Cholesterol: 51 milligrams

Protein: 37 grams

Sodium: 419 milligrams

Calcium: 163 milligrams

Added sugar: 0 grams

INCLUDES THE FOLLOWING SERVINGS
FROM THE FOOD GROUPS:

Protein: 5 servings

Vegetables: 1 serving

Black Bean Burgers with Horseradish Mayonnaise

Serves 6

Black beans are rich in soluble fiber, which helps to reduce blood cholesterol and fosters normal blood glucose levels. Quinoa is a quick-cooking protein-rich whole grain that also supplies fiber and holds these meatless burgers together! These are served on whole-wheat rolls with a horseradish mayonnaise, but you could also serve in pita pockets or alongside a large salad and skip the rolls.

4 garlic cloves, roughly chopped

1 (15-ounce) can black beans, drained and rinsed

2 tablespoons tomato paste

1 teaspoon ground cumin

1 teaspoon salt

½ teaspoon paprika

1 teaspoon ground chipotle chile pepper

1 tablespoon Worcestershire sauce

2 large eggs

¼ cup drained and chopped jarred roasted red peppers, in ¼-inch pieces

1½ cups cooked quinoa

½ cup panko bread crumbs

2 tablespoons canola oil

6 whole-wheat burger rolls, about 2 ounces each

HORSERADISH MAYONNAISE

Makes 4 tablespoons

2 tablespoons reduced-fat mayonnaise

2 tablespoons prepared horseradish

Freshly ground black pepper

1. Place the garlic, beans, tomato paste, cumin, salt, paprika, chipotle chile pepper, and Worcestershire sauce in a food processor and process until the mixture becomes a paste, 30 to 45 seconds. Transfer to a medium mixing bowl, then add the eggs, red peppers, quinoa, and bread crumbs. Mix well. Form the mixture into 6 equal-size patties.

2. In a large nonstick skillet or grill pan, heat the oil over medium-high heat. Add the patties and reduce the heat to medium. Cook the patties for 5 to 7 minutes on each side, until lightly browned.

3. Prepare the Horseradish Mayonnaise by combining all the ingredients in a small bowl.

4. Place burgers on rolls and top with mayonnaise.

**PER SERVING (WITH ROLL AND
2 TEASPOONS MAYONNAISE):**

Calories: 240

Carbohydrate: 29 grams

Dietary fiber: 7 grams

Total fat: 10 grams

Saturated fat: 1 gram

Cholesterol: 64 milligrams

Protein: 9 grams

Sodium: 526 milligrams

Calcium: 59 milligrams

Added sugar: 0 grams

**INCLUDES THE FOLLOWING SERVINGS
FROM THE FOOD GROUPS:**

Grains: ½ serving

Protein: about 1 serving

Vegetables: ½ serving

Simple Meals for When Time Is Tight

When we get busy, meal planning goes out the window, and we're assuming it's the same for you. That's why it's important to have healthy, convenient ingredients on hand to make meals in a flash. Here are some of our favorite "fast-food" ideas for one meal. You can double or quadruple the recipes as needed.

(continued)

- Spread 2 slices of whole-grain bread with 2 tablespoons sunflower seed butter and top with 1 sliced small banana or 2 tablespoons raisins. Serve with 8 ounces of 1% low-fat dairy milk or fortified unsweetened soy milk, and fruit.
- Scramble 2 eggs and divide between halves of a small whole-wheat pita round. Add salsa, ½ cup raw baby spinach, and ¼ cup shredded cheddar cheese. Serve with 8 ounces dairy milk or fortified soy milk.
- One hard-cooked egg, ½ cup plain fat-free Greek yogurt, 1 slice of whole-grain toast, and fruit.
- In a bowl, layer 1 cup cooked whole grains, such as quinoa, farro, or brown rice, with 1 cup cooked vegetables and at least 3 ounces of tofu or cooked salmon or chicken.

SIDE DISHES

Farro Salad with Golden Raisins and Pistachios

Serves 4

Farro is a whole grain that's rich in fiber, protein, and phytonutrients. Add chopped cooked chicken to make this a meal.

1 cup pearled farro

2 tablespoons fresh lemon juice

1 tablespoon olive oil

½ teaspoon salt

½ teaspoon freshly ground black pepper

¼ cup golden raisins

¼ cup chopped shelled pistachios

1. Cook the farro according to package directions. Transfer to a mixing bowl to cool for about 20 minutes.
2. In a small bowl, whisk together the lemon juice, oil, salt, and pepper until well blended.
3. Add the raisins to the farro, drizzle on the dressing, and mix well. Top with the pistachios and serve.

PER SERVING:

Calories: 280

Carbohydrate: 47 grams

Dietary fiber: 8 grams

Total fat: 8 grams

Saturated fat: 1 gram

Cholesterol: 0 milligrams

Protein: 9 grams

Sodium: 299 milligrams

Calcium: 22 milligrams

Added sugar: 0 grams

INCLUDES THE FOLLOWING SERVINGS FROM THE FOOD GROUPS:

Grains: ½ serving

Protein: 1 serving

Golden Roasted Cauliflower

Serves 4

Say good-bye to boring vegetables! Turmeric and paprika spice up this roasted cauliflower dish in more ways than one.

1 large head or 2 small heads of cauliflower, trimmed and cut into florets

3 tablespoons olive oil

2 teaspoons garlic powder

½ teaspoon ground turmeric

½ teaspoon paprika

½ teaspoon salt

1. Preheat the oven to 400°F. Coat a large baking sheet with cooking spray.
2. Place the cauliflower florets in a large bowl.
3. In a small bowl, whisk together the oil, garlic powder, turmeric, paprika, and salt. Pour evenly over the cauliflower and toss well to coat all the pieces.
4. Spread the cauliflower on the baking sheet and roast for 10 minutes. Remove the baking sheet from the oven, stir the cauliflower, and return to the oven for another 10 to 15 minutes, or until the florets are fork-tender and caramelized.

PER SERVING:

Calories: 160

Carbohydrate: 14 grams

Dietary fiber: 6 grams

Total fat: 11 grams

Saturated fat: 2 grams

Cholesterol: 0 milligrams

Protein: 5 grams

Sodium: 380 milligrams

Calcium: 63 milligrams

Added sugar: 0 grams

INCLUDES THE FOLLOWING SERVINGS FROM THE FOOD GROUPS:

Vegetables: 1 serving

SNACKS AND DESSERTS

Creamy Chocolate Peanut Butter "Ice Cream"

Serves 2

Here is a frozen fruit-based treat that simultaneously tackles cravings for ice cream, peanut butter, and chocolate, and without added sugar!

2 medium-ripe bananas, cut into chunks and frozen (at least 2 hours)

2 tablespoons natural peanut butter (without added sugar, if desired)

2 tablespoons unsweetened cocoa powder

½ teaspoon vanilla extract

2 tablespoons chopped peanuts

1. Place the bananas in a food processor or blender. Add the peanut butter, cocoa powder, and vanilla. Blend until smooth, 2 to 3 minutes.
2. Transfer to serving bowls and garnish with the peanuts. Serve immediately.

PER SERVING:

Calories: 251

Carbohydrate: 32 grams

Dietary fiber: 5 grams

Total fat: 13 grams

Saturated fat: 2 grams

Cholesterol: 0 milligrams

Protein: 8 grams

Sodium: 4 milligrams

Calcium: 24 milligrams

Added sugar: 0 grams

**INCLUDES THE FOLLOWING SERVINGS
FROM THE FOOD GROUPS:**
Fruit: 1 serving
Protein: 1 serving

Chocolate Oatmeal Energy Balls

Makes 20 balls

Most energy balls aren't high enough in protein for our purposes, so we made our own using protein powder. And yes, with honey (or syrup) because you need something to hold all the ingredients together!

¾ **cup natural peanut butter (without added sugar, if desired)**

½ **cup honey or maple syrup**

⅔ **cup chocolate whey protein powder**

1 **teaspoon vanilla extract**

2½ **cups quick or old-fashioned rolled oats**

1. Place the peanut butter in microwave-safe dish. Microwave for 30 to 40 seconds, or until melted. Place the melted peanut butter in a large mixing bowl.
2. Add the honey, protein powder, and vanilla, and stir until completely combined. Add the oats and stir again to combine well.
3. Form the mixture into 20 balls. (Store in an airtight container in the refrigerator or freezer.)

PER SERVING (2 BALLS):
Calories: 264
Carbohydrate: 33 grams
Dietary fiber: 4 grams

Total fat: 12 grams
Saturated fat: 2 grams
Cholesterol: 10 milligrams

Protein: 11 grams   Calcium: 58 milligrams
Sodium: 101 milligrams   Added sugar: 14 grams

INCLUDES THE FOLLOWING SERVINGS
FROM THE FOOD GROUPS:
Grains: ½ serving
Protein: 1½ servings

Roasted Strawberries with Greek Yogurt

Serves 2

We love all types of berries, but strawberries are particularly good for roasting because they hold up well to heat.

1 quart fresh strawberries (about 3½ cups), washed, hulled, and halved lengthwise

1 tablespoon sugar

1 teaspoon vanilla extract

1 cup plain fat-free Greek yogurt

1. Preheat the oven to 375°F. Line a large baking sheet with parchment paper.
2. Place the strawberries in a medium bowl. Add the sugar and vanilla, and toss to combine well.
3. Spread the strawberries on the baking sheet and roast in the oven for 20 to 25 minutes, or until the strawberries are fork-tender.
4. Let the strawberries cool for 5 minutes on the baking sheet, then transfer them along with any juices to a container. (Refrigerate if not using right away.)

5. To serve, place ½ cup of yogurt in each bowl and top each with half the strawberries and their juices.

PER SERVING:

Calories: 169

Carbohydrate: 28 grams

Dietary fiber: 5 grams

Total fat: 1 gram

Saturated fat: 0 grams

Cholesterol: 6 milligrams

Protein: 14 grams

Sodium: 46 milligrams

Calcium: 171 milligrams

Added sugar: 6 grams

INCLUDES THE FOLLOWING SERVINGS FROM THE FOOD GROUPS:

Dairy: ½ serving

Fruit: 1 serving

Protein: 2 servings

Cherry Frozen Yogurt

Serves 2

Yogurt with active cultures is a source of probiotics—living organisms that help keep the gut healthy. Eating yogurt on a regular basis may promote healthier blood pressure, too.[5] Add 2 tablespoons dark chocolate chips or cocoa nibs to the mix, if desired.

2 cups frozen pitted sweet cherries

¼ cup 1% low-fat milk

½ cup plain fat-free Greek yogurt

1 teaspoon vanilla extract

1. Combine all the ingredients in a blender or food processor and blend on high speed until smooth.
2. Enjoy immediately or store in a container in the freezer.

PER SERVING:

Calories: 137

Carbohydrate: 26 grams

Dietary fiber: 3 grams

Total fat: 1 gram

Saturated fat: 0 grams

Cholesterol: 5 milligrams

Protein: 9 grams

Sodium: 36 milligrams

Calcium: 124 milligrams

Added sugar: 0 grams

INCLUDES THE FOLLOWING SERVINGS FROM THE FOOD GROUPS:

Dairy: ½ serving

Fruit: 1 serving

Protein: about 1 serving

RESOURCES

GENERAL MENOPAUSE INFORMATION

U.S. Department of Health and Human Services
Office on Women's Health
https://www.womenshealth.gov/menopause/menopause-resources

American College of Obstetricians and Gynecologists
https://www.acog.org/patients

The North American Menopause Society
https://www.menopause.org/for-women

U.S. Food and Drug Administration
Menopause
https://www.fda.gov/consumers/womens-health-topics/menopause

The National Library of Medicine
Menopause
https://bit.ly/2oeWpUB

Hormone Health Network
https://www.hormone.org/your-health-and-hormones/womens-health

PHYSICAL ACTIVITY AND EXERCISE

Move Your Way Activity Planner
https://health.gov/MoveYourWay/Activity-Planner/

DIETARY SUPPLEMENTS

National Institutes of Health
Dietary Supplement Label Database
https://www.dsld.nlm.nih.gov/dsld/

National Institutes of Health, Office of Dietary Supplements
https://ods.od.nih.gov/

About Herbs, Botanicals and Other Products, Memorial Sloan Kettering
    Cancer Center
https://www.mskcc.org/cancer-care/diagnosis-treatment/symptom
    -management/integrative-medicine/herbs

RECOMMENDED READING

*The Prediabetes Diet Plan: How to Reverse Prediabetes and Prevent
    Diabetes through Healthy Eating and Exercise,* by Hillary Wright.
*The PCOS Diet Plan: A Natural Approach to Health for Women with
    Polycystic Ovary Syndrome,* by Hillary Wright.
*The Type 2 Diabetic Cookbook and Action Plan: A Three-Month Kickstart
    Guide for Living Well with Type 2 Diabetes,* by Martha McKittrick.
*The Wisdom of Menopause: Creating Physical and Emotional Health
    During the Change,* by Christiane Northrup.
Eat Out, Eat Well: The Guide to Healthy Eating in Any Restaurant, by
    Hope Warshaw.

Food and Fitness After 50: Eat Well, Move Well, Be Well, by Christine
  Rosenbloom and Bob Murray.
*The DASH Diet Mediterranean Solution: The Best Eating Plan to Control
  Your Weight and Improve Your Health for Life*, by Marla Heller.
DASH Diet for Dummies, by Sarah Samann, Rosanne Rust, and Cindy
  Kleckner.
*The MIND Diet: A Scientific Approach to Enhancing Brain Function and
  Helping Prevent Alzheimer's and Dementia*, by Maggie Moon.
Intuitive Eating: A Revolutionary Program That Works, by Evelyn Tribole
  and Elyse Resch.
Our Bodies, Ourselves: Menopause, by Boston Women's Health Collective
  and Judy Norsigian.
*Mindful Eating: A Guide to Rediscovering a Healthy and Joyful
  Relationship with Food*, by Jan Chozen Bays.

HEALTHY WAYS TO EAT

MyPlate
https://www.choosemyplate.gov

New American Plate
https://www.aicr.org/new-american-plate/

Healthy Eating Plate
https://www.hsph.harvard.edu/nutritionsource/healthy-eating-plate/

GENERAL NUTRITION INFORMATION

Center for Science in the Public Interest
https://www.cspinet.org

Harvard School of Public Health Nutrition Source
https://www.hsph.harvard.edu/nutritionsource/

HEALTHY COOKING MAGAZINES

Cooking Light
https://www.cookinglight.com

Eating Well
https://www.eatingwell.com

USEFUL TOOLS FOR TRACKING CALORIES AND PHYSICAL ACTIVITY

SelfNutritionData
https://nutritiondata.self.com/

Good Measures
https://www.goodmeasures.com

MyFitnessPal
https://www.myfitnesspal.com

MyNetDiary
https://www.mynetdiary.com

ACKNOWLEDGMENTS

Without the support and encouragement of so many people, this book never would have come to be. We'd like to thank our agent, Judith Riven, for her guidance and wisdom, and our editor Michele Eniclerico and the staff at Harmony/Rodale for helping to improve on our work. A special shout-out to the very talented David Parmentier for producing beautiful visuals and his patience with us as we communicated our vision. Thank you to all of our colleagues who saw the value in what we were creating and cheered us on. Your support was invaluable in keeping the ball rolling. And, to our village of women family members and friends—and countless patients over the years—who rode the menopause wave before us, thanks for the advice and for sharing your experiences. Your guidance helped us both personally and professionally to navigate this phase of life.

HILLARY

I'm fortunate to have a large, loving family who have always been my biggest fans. I'd like to thank my parents, Alan and Marie Wright, my cheering section for all things in life; my in-laws Nancy and Jack

Holowitz (and the rest of the Holowitz/Parmentier clan!), for your support and pride in my work; my sister Alison and my brothers John, Chris, Brian, and Michael, and their families; and my husband, Tony, and my beautiful sons—John, Matthew, and Brian—thanks so much for helping me make room in my life for my writing. I love you. And, of course, thank you Liz. My dear friend for so long, and now my partner in crime. Watch out world!

LIZ

They say it takes a village, and when you're writing a book, that's certainly true. Thanks to my husband, Tom, and our three wonderful daughters—Hayley, Hannah, and Emma—for tolerating me during the writing and editing process, especially when I may have been a bit cranky. I couldn't have done it without you! And thanks to Hillary, who always pushes me to be a better writer, a more considerate health professional, and a better person.

REFERENCES

CHAPTER 1

1. Sacks FM, et al. DASH-Sodium Collaborative Research Group. Effects on blood pressure of reduced dietary sodium and the Dietary Approaches to Stop Hypertension (DASH) diet. *N Engl J Med.* January 2001; 344(1):3–10.
2. Saneei P, et al. Influence of Dietary Approaches to Stop Hypertension (DASH) diet on blood pressure: a systematic review and meta-analysis on randomized controlled trials. *Nutr Metab Cardiovasc Dis.* December 2014; 24(12):1253–61.
3. Sayon-Orea C, et al. Adherence to Mediterranean dietary pattern and menopausal symptoms in relation to overweight/obesity in Spanish perimenopausal and postmenopausal women. *Menopause.* July 2015; 22(7):750–57.
4. Liu ZM, et al. Whole plant foods intake is associated with fewer menopausal symptoms in Chinese postmenopausal women with prehypertension or untreated hypertension. *Menopause.* May 2015; 22(5):496–504.
5. Ford C, et al. Evaluation of diet pattern and weight gain in postmenopausal women enrolled in the Women's Health Initiative Observational Study. *Br J Nutr.* April 2017; 117(8):1189–97.

CHAPTER 2

1. U.S. Department of Health and Human Services. National Institutes of Health. National Institute of Diabetes and Digestive and Kidney Diseases. Available at https://www.niddk.nih.gov/health-information/health-statistics/overweight -obesity.

2. Kapoor E, et al. Weight gain in women at midlife: a concise review of the pathophysiology and strategies for management. *Mayo Clin Proc.* October 2017; 92(10):1552–58.

3. Anderson LJ, et al. Sex differences in muscle wasting. *Adv Exp Med Biol.* December 10, 2017; 1043:153–97.

4. Study of Women's Health Across the Nation. Changes in body composition and weight during the menopause transition. Available at https://www.swanstudy.org/changes-in-body-composition-and-weight-during-the-menopause-transition/.

5. Davis SR, et al. Understanding weight gain at menopause. *Climacteric.* October 2012; 15:419–29.

6. Cleary MP & Grossman ME. Obesity and breast cancer: the estrogen connection. *Endocrinology.* June 2009; 150(6):2537–42.

7. Centers for Disease Control and Prevention. Diabetes prevention. Available at https://www.cdc.gov/diabetes/prevention/index.html.

8. U.S. Department of Health and Human Services. National Heart, Lung, and Blood Institute. Overweight and obesity. Available at https://www.nhlbi.nih.gov/health-topics/overweight-and-obesity.

9. Teachman J. Body weight, marital status, and changes in marital status. *Journal of Family Issues.* January 1, 2016; 37(1):74–96.

10. U.S. Department of Health and Human Services. National Heart, Lung, and Blood Institute. Overweight and obesity. Available at https://www.nhlbi.nih.gov/health-topics/overweight-and-obesity.

11. Jung SY, et al. Risk profiles for weight gain among postmenopausal women: a classification and regression tree analysis approach. *PLoS One.* March 20, 2015; 10(3): e0121430.

12. Stachowiak G, et al. Metabolic disorders in menopause. *Prz Menopauzalny.* March 2015; 14:59–64.

13. Schreiber DR & Dautovich ND. Depressive symptoms and weight in midlife women: the role of stress eating and menopause status. *Menopause.* October 2017; 24(10):1190–99.

14. National Weight Control Registry. Available at http://www.nwcr.ws/default.htm.

15. Lillis J, et al. Internal disinhibition predicts five-year weight regain in the National Weight Control Registry (NWCR). *Obes Sci Pract.* March 2016; 2(1):83–87.

16. Ross KM, et al. Successful weight loss maintenance associated with morning chronotype and better sleep quality. *J Behav Med.* June 2016; 39(3):465–71.

17. Thomas JG, et al. Weight-loss maintenance for ten years in the National Weight Control Registry. *Am J Prev Med.* 2014; 46(1):17–23.

18. Manoogian ENC & Panda S. Circadian rhythms, time-restricted feeding, and healthy aging. *Ageing Res Rev.* October 2017; 39:59–67.

19. Stenvers DJ, et al. Circadian clocks and insulin resistance. *Nat Rev Endocrinol.* February 2019; 15(2):75–89.

20. Jacobowicz D, et al. High caloric intake at breakfast vs. dinner differentially influences weight loss of overweight and obese women. *Obesity.* December 2013; 21(12):2504–12.

21. Jackson KL, et al. Body image satisfaction and depression in midlife women: the Study of Women's Health Across the Nation (SWAN). *Arch Womens Ment Health.* June 2014; 17(3):177–87.

CHAPTER 3

1. McSweeney JC, et al. Preventing and experiencing ischemic heart disease as a woman: state of the science: a scientific statement from the American Heart Association. *Circulation.* March 2016; 133(13):1302–31.
2. Mehta LS, et al. Acute myocardial infarction in women: a scientific statement from the American Heart Association. *Circulation.* March 2016; 133(9):916–47.
3. Johns Hopkins Medicine. Peripheral Vascular Disease. Available at https://www.hopkinsmedicine.org/healthlibrary/conditions/cardiovascular_diseases/peripheral_vascular_disease_85,p00236.
4. U.S. Department of Health and Human Services, National Heart, Lung, and Blood Institute. Ischemic heart disease. Available at https://www.nhlbi.nih.gov/health-topics/ischemic-heart-disease.
5. Ibid.
6. Muka T, et al. Association of age at onset of menopause and time since onset of menopause with cardiovascular outcomes, intermediate vascular traits, and all-cause mortality: a systematic review and meta-analysis. *JAMA Cardiol.* October 2016; 1(7):767–76.
7. Lisabeth LD, et al. Age at natural menopause and risk of ischemic stroke: the Framingham Heart Study. *Stroke.* April 2009; 40(4):1044–49.
8. Cleveland Clinic. Women and abnormal heartbeats. Available at https://my.clevelandclinic.org/health/diseases/17644-women-abnormal-heart-beats.
9. U.S. Department of Health and Human Services, National Heart, Lung, and Blood Institute. Ischemic heart disease. Available at https://www.nhlbi.nih.gov/health-topics/ischemic-heart-disease.
10. Peters SAE, et al. Sex differences in the association between measures of general and central adiposity and the risk of myocardial infarction: results from the UK biobank. *J Am Heart Assoc.* March 2018; 7(5):1–12.
11. Huo X, et al. Risk of non-fatal cardiovascular diseases in early-onset versus late-onset type 2 diabetes in China: a cross-sectional study. *Lancet Diabetes Endocrinol.* February 2016; 4(2):115–24.
12. Huang Y, et al. Association between prediabetes and risk of cardiovascular disease and all causes mortality: systematic review and meta-analysis. *BMJ.* November 2016; 355:i5953.
13. Taddei S. Blood pressure through aging and menopause. *Climacteric.* September 2009; 12 Suppl 1; 36–40.
14. U.S. Department of Health and Human Services, National Institute of Aging. High blood pressure. Available at https://www.nia.nih.gov/health/high-blood-pressure.

15. American Heart Association. What your cholesterol levels mean. Available at https://www.heart.org/en/health-topics/cholesterol/about-cholesterol/what-your -cholesterol-levels-mean.

16. U.S. Department of Health and Human Services. National Heart, Lung, and Blood Institute. High blood cholesterol. Available at https://www.nhlbi.nih.gov /health-topics/high-blood-cholesterol.

17. U.S. Department of Health and Human Services. National Heart, Lung, and Blood Institute. High blood triglycerides. Available at https://www.nhlbi.nih.gov /health-topics/high-blood-triglycerides.

18. Sacks FM, et al. on behalf of the American Heart Association. Dietary fats and cardiovascular disease: a presidential advisory from the American Heart Association. *Circulation.* July 2017; 136(3):e1–e23.

19. U.S. Department of Health and Human Services, National Heart, Lung, and Blood Institute. Smoking and your heart. Available at www.nhlbi.nih.gov /health-topics/smoking-and-your-heart.

20. U.S. Department of Health and Human Services. Physical activity guidelines for Americans, 2nd edition. 2018. Available at https://health.gov/paguidelines /second-edition/.

21. Watson NF, et al. Recommended amount of sleep for a healthy adult: a joint consensus statement of the American Academy of Sleep Medicine and Sleep Research Society. *J Clin Sleep Med.* 2015; 11(6):591–92.

22. Vahratian A. Sleep duration and quality among women aged 40–59, by menopausal status. *NCHS Data Brief.* September 2017; (286):1–8.

23. U.S. Department of Health and Human Services. National Heart, Lung, and Blood Institute. Sleep deprivation and deficiency. Available at https://www.nhlbi .nih.gov/health-topics/sleep-deprivation-and-deficiency.

24. U.S. Department of Health and Human Services, National Institute for Aging. A good night's sleep. Available at https://www.nia.nih.gov/health/good-nights -sleep.

25. U.S. Department of Health and Human Services. National Heart, Lung, and Blood Institute. Insomnia. Available at https://www.nhlbi.nih.gov/health-topics /insomnia.

26. U.S. Department of Health and Human Services. Physical activity guidelines for Americans, 2nd edition. 2018. Available at https://health.gov/paguidelines /second-edition/.

27. American Heart Association. Fish and omega-3 fatty acids. Available at https:// www.heart.org/en/healthy-living/healthy-eating/eat-smart/fats/fish-and-omega-3 -fatty-acids.

28. U.S. Department of Health and Human Services. National Institutes of Health. Office of Dietary Supplements. Omega-3 fatty acids. Available at https://ods.od .nih.gov/factsheets/Omega3FattyAcids-HealthProfessional/.

29. U.S. Department of Health and Human Services & U.S. Department of Agriculture. Dietary guidelines for Americans 2015–2020, 8th edition. A closer look inside

eating patterns. Available at https://health.gov/dietaryguidelines/2015/guidelines/chapter-1/a-closer-look-inside-healthy-eating-patterns/#callout-seafood.

30. Thompson M, et al. Omega-3 fatty acid intake by age, gender, and pregnancy status in the United States: National Health and Nutrition Examination Survey 2003–2014. *Nutrients.* January 15, 2019; 11(1):177.

31. Eckel RH, et al. 2013 AHA/ACC guideline on lifestyle management to reduce cardiovascular risk: a report of the American College of Cardiology/American Heart Association Task Force on Practice Guidelines. *J Am Coll Cardio.* 2014; 63:2960–84.

32. Ibid.

33. Reynolds A, et al. Carbohydrate quality and human health: a series of systematic reviews and meta-analyses. *Lancet.* February 2019; 393(10170):434–45.

34. Centers for Disease Control and Prevention. Get the facts: sodium and the dietary guidelines. Available at https://www.cdc.gov/salt/pdfs/sodium_dietary_guidelines.pdf.

35. Maluly H, et al. Monosodium glutamate as a tool to reduce sodium in foodstuffs: technological and safety aspects. *Food Sci Nutr.* July 2017; 5(6):1039–48.

36. National Academies of Sciences, Engineering, and Medicine. *Dietary Reference Intakes for Sodium and Potassium.* Washington, DC: National Academies Press, 2019.

37. U.S. Department of Health and Human Services. National Institutes of Health. Office of Dietary Supplements. Magnesium. Available at https://ods.od.nih.gov/factsheets/Magnesium-HealthProfessional/#en42.

38. Kopecky SL, et al. Lack of evidence linking calcium with or without vitamin D supplementation to cardiovascular disease in generally healthy adults: a clinical guideline from the national osteoporosis foundation and the American Society for Preventive Cardiology. *Ann Intern Med.* October 2016; (165):867–68.

CHAPTER 4

1. Centers for Disease Control and Prevention. National diabetes statistics report, 2017. Available at https://www.cdc.gov/diabetes/data/statistics-report/index.html.

2. Centers for Disease Control and Prevention. CDC diabetes infographics. Available at https://www.cdc.gov/diabetes/library/socialMedia/infographics.html.

3. Heianza Y, et al. Effect of postmenopausal status and age at menopause on type 2 diabetes and prediabetes in Japanese individuals: Toranomon Hospital Health Management Center Study 17 (TOPICS 17). *Diabetes Care.* December 2013; 36(12):4007–14.

4. Muka T, et al. Age at natural menopause and risk of type 2 diabetes: a prospective cohort study. *Diabetologia.* October 2017; 60(10):1951–60.

5. Centers for Disease Control and Prevention. Leading causes of death—females-all

races and origins—United States, 2017. Available at https://www.cdc.gov/women/lcod/2017/all-races-origins/index.htm.

6. Moheet A, et al. Impact of diabetes on cognitive function and brain structure. *Ann NY Acad Sci.* September 2015; 1353:60–71.

7. Nathan DM, et al. Impaired fasting glucose and impaired glucose tolerance: implications for care. *Diabetes Care.* March 2007; 30(3):753–59.

8. Slopian R, et al. Menopause and diabetes: EMAS clinical guide. *Maturitas.* November 2018; 117:6–10.

9. Centers for Disease Control and Prevention. Diabetes: who's at risk. Available at https://www.cdc.gov/diabetes/basics/risk-factors.html.

10. Bruno Ade S, et al. Non-alcoholic fatty liver disease and its associated risk factors in Brazilian postmenopausal women. *Climacteric.* August 2014; 17(4):465–71.

11. American Diabetes Association. Diagnosing diabetes and learning about prediabetes. Available at http://diabetes.org/diabetes-basics/diagnosis/.

12. Alexander CM, et al. NCEP-defined metabolic syndrome, diabetes, and prevalence of coronary heart disease among NHANES III participants age 50 years and older. *Diabetes.* May 2003; 52(5):1210–14, https://diabetes.diabetesjournals.org/content/52/5/1210.

13. American Heart Association. What is metabolic syndrome? Available at https://www.heart.org/-/media/files/health-topics/answers-by-heart/what-is-metabolic-syndrome-300322.pdf?la=en&hash=3B60478685B71C2CD6CEB93782DAE8B7EAD33445.

14. American Heart Association. About metabolic syndrome. Available at https://www.heart.org/en/health-topics/metabolic-syndrome/about-metabolic-syndrome.

15. U.S. National Library of Medicine. Medline Plus: metabolic syndrome. Available at https://medlineplus.gov/ency/article/007290.htm.

16. Mottillo S, et al. The metabolic syndrome and cardiovascular risk: a systematic review and meta-analysis. *J Am Coll Cardio.* September 2010; 56(14):1113–32.

17. U.S. Department of Health and Human Services. Office on Women's Health. Polycystic ovary syndrome. Available at https://www.womenshealth.gov/a-z-topics/polycystic-ovary-syndrome.

18. Wright H. *The PCOS Diet Plan: A Natural Approach to Health for Women with Polycystic Ovary Syndrome.* New York: Penguin Random House, 2019.

19. Diabetes Prevention Program. Reduction in the incidence of type 2 diabetes with lifestyle intervention or metformin. *N Engl J Med.* February 7, 2002; 346:393–403.

20. Reaven G. The metabolic syndrome: is this diagnosis necessary? *Am J Clin Nutr.* June 2006; 83(6):1237–47.

21. Harvard Health Publishing. Eating too much added sugar increases the risk of dying with heart disease. Available at https://www.health.harvard.edu/blog/eating-too-much-added-sugar-increases-the-risk-of-dying-with-heart-disease-201402067021.

22. Jannasch F, et al. Dietary patterns and type 2 diabetes: a systematic literature review and meta-analysis of prospective studies. *J Nutr.* June 2017; 147(6):1174–82.

23. Diabetes Education Services. Available at https://diabetesed.net/page/_files/THE-DIABETIC-EXCHANGE-LIST.pdf.

24. Hughes VA. Exercise increases muscle GLUT-4 levels and insulin action in subjects with impaired glucose tolerance. *Am J Physiol.* June 1992; 264(6 part 1): E855–62.

25. Tuomilehto, J. Nonpharmacologic therapy and exercise in the prevention of type 2 diabetes. *Diabetes Care.* November 2009; 32:S189–93.

CHAPTER 5

1. Jacobs EG, et al. Impact of sex and menopausal status on episodic memory circuitry in early midlife. *J Neuroscience.* September 2016; 36(39):10163–73.

2. Mosconi L, et al. Perimenopause and emergence of an Alzheimer's bioenergetic phenotype in brain and periphery. *PLoS ONE.* October 2017; 12(10):e0185926.

3. Epperson CN, et al. Menopause effects on verbal memory: findings from a longitudinal community cohort. *J Clin Endocrinol Metab.* September 2013; 98(9):3829–38.

4. Greendale GA, et al. Effects of the menopause transition and hormone use on cognitive performance in midlife women. *Neurology.* May 2009; 72(21):1850–57.

5. Echouffo-Tcheugui JB, et al. Circulating cortisol and cognitive and structural brain measures. *Neurology.* November 2018; 91(21):e1961–70.

6. Hall MH, et al. Chronic stress is prospectively associated with sleep in midlife women: the SWAN Sleep Study. *Sleep.* October 2015; 38(10):1645–54.

7. National Institutes of Health. National Institute for Mental Health. Anxiety disorders. Available at https://www.nimh.nih.gov/health/topics/anxiety-disorders/index.shtml.

8. Centers for Disease Control and Prevention. Mental health conditions: depression and anxiety. Available at https://www.cdc.gov/tobacco/campaign/tips/diseases/depression-anxiety.html#three.

9. National Institutes of Health. National Institute for Mental Health. Depression. Available at https://www.nimh.nih.gov/health/topics/anxiety-disorders/index.shtml.

10. Bromberger JT & Kravitz HM. Mood and menopause: findings from the Study of Women's Health Across the Nation (SWAN) over 10 years. *Obstet Gynecol Clin North Am.* September 2011; 38(3):609–25.

11. Bromberger JT, et al. Longitudinal change in reproductive hormones and depressive symptoms across the menopausal transition: results from the Study of Women's Health Across the Nation (SWAN). *Arch Gen Psychiatry.* June 2010; 67(6):598–607.

12. National Institutes of Health. National Institute on Aging. Depression and older adults. Available at https://www.nia.nih.gov/health/depression-and-older-adults.

13. Lisabeth LD, et al. Age at natural menopause and risk of ischemic stroke: the Framingham Heart Study. *Stroke.* April 2009; 40(4):1044–49.

14. American Heart Association. How high blood pressure can lead to stroke. Available at https://www.heart.org/en/health-topics/high-blood-pressure/health -threats-from-high-blood-pressure/how-high-blood-pressure-can-lead-to-stroke.

15. Mayo Clinic. Transient ischemic attack. Available at https://www.mayoclinic.org /diseases-conditions/transient-ischemic-attack/symptoms-causes/syc-20355679.

16. American Stroke Association. American stroke month. Available at https:// www.strokeassociation.org/en/about-the-american-stroke-association/american -stroke-month.

17. Centers for Disease Control and Prevention. Smoking and heart disease and stroke. Available at https://www.cdc.gov/tobacco/campaign/tips/diseases/heart -disease-stroke.html.

18. National Institutes of Health. National Institute on Aging. What is dementia? Symptoms, types, and diagnosis. Available at https://www.nia.nih.gov/health /what-dementia-symptoms-types-and-diagnosis.

19. den Heijer T, et al. A 10-year follow-up of hippocampal volume on magnetic resonance imaging in early dementia and cognitive decline. *Brain.* April 2010; 133(4):1163–72.

20. Morris MC, et al. MIND diet associated with reduced incidence of Alzheimer's disease. *Alzheimers Dement.* September 2015; 11(9):1007–14.

21. Valls-Pedret C, et al. Mediterranean diet and age-related cognitive decline: a randomized clinical trial. *JAMA Intern Med.* July 2015; 175(7):1094–103.

22. Blumenthal JA, et al. Lifestyle and neurocognition in older adults with cognitive impairments. *Neurology.* January 2019; 92(3):e212–23.

23. Lourida I, et al. Association of lifestyle and genetic risk with incidence of dementia. *JAMA.* July 14, 2019; 322(5):430–37.

24. Tan ZS, et al. Red blood cell ω-3 fatty acid levels and markers of accelerated brain aging. *Neurology.* February 2012; 78(9):658–64.

25. Pottala JV, et al. Higher RBC, EPA + DHA corresponds with larger total brain and hippocampal volumes: WHIMS-MRI study. *Neurology.* February 2014; 82(5):435–42.

26. Zhang Y, et al. Intakes of fish and polyunsaturated fatty acids and mild-to-severe cognitive impairment risks: a dose-response meta-analysis of 21 cohort studies. *Am J Clin Nutr.* February 2016; 103(2):330–40.

27. Li F, et al. Fish consumption and risk of depression: a meta-analysis *J Epidemiol Community Health.* March 2016; 70(3):299–304.

28. U.S. Department of Health and Human Services & U.S. Department of Agriculture. Dietary guidelines for Americans 2015–2020. 8th edition. A closer look inside eating patterns. Available at https://health.gov/dietaryguidelines/2015/guidelines /chapter-1/a-closer-look-inside-healthy-eating-patterns/#callout-seafood.

29. Poly C, et al. The relation of dietary choline to cognitive performance and white-

matter hyperintensity in the Framingham Offspring Cohort. *Am J Clin Nutr.* December 2011; 94(6):1584–91.

30. Blusztain JK, et al. Neuroprotective actions of dietary choline. *Nutrients.* July 28, 2017; 9(8):815.

31. U.S. Department of Agriculture, Agricultural Research Service, Food Surveys Research Group. What we eat in America data tables. Available at https://www.ars.usda.gov/northeast-area/beltsville-md-bhnrc/beltsville-human-nutrition-research-center/food-surveys-research-group/docs/wweia-data-tables/.

32. Fischer LM, et al. Dietary choline requirements of women: effects of estrogen and genetic variation. *Am J Clin Nutr.* November 2010; 92(5):1113–19.

33. U.S. Department of Health and Human Services. National Institutes of Health. Office of Dietary Supplements. Vitamin B_{12}. Available at https://ods.od.nih.gov/factsheets/VitaminB12-HealthProfessional/.

34. Johnson EJ. Role of lutein and zeaxanthin in visual and cognitive function throughout the lifespan. *Nutrition Reviews.* September 1, 2014; 72(9): 605–12.

35. Boespflug EL & Iliff JJ. The emerging relationship between interstitial fluid-cerebrospinal fluid exchange, amyloid-β, and sleep. *Biol Psychiatry.* February 2018; 83(4):328–36.

36. Varga AW, et al. Apnea-induced rapid eye movement sleep disruption impairs human spatial navigational memory. *J Neuroscience.* October 29, 2014; 34(44):14571–77.

37. Coupland CAC, et al. Anticholinergic drug exposure and the risk of dementia: a nested case-control study. *JAMA Intern Med.* 2019; 179(8):1084–93.

38. U.S. Food and Drug Administration. FDA drug safety communication: important safety label changes to cholesterol-lowering statin drugs. Available at https://www.fda.gov/drugs/drug-safety-and-availability/fda-drug-safety-communication-important-safety-label-changes-cholesterol-lowering-statin-drugs.

39. Rehm J. Alcohol use and dementia: a systematic scoping review. *Alzheimers Res Ther.* January 2019; 11(1):1. Available at https://alzres.biomedcentral.com/articles/10.1186/s13195-018-0453-0.

40. Cook AH, et al. Psychological well-being in elderly adults with extraordinary episodic memory. *PLoS ONE.* 2017; 12(10):e0186413.

CHAPTER 6

1. American Institute for Cancer Research. Can cancer be prevented? Available at https://www.aicr.org/reduce-your-cancer-risk/smoking-and-other-lifestyle-factors/cancer-prevention.html.

2. National Cancer Institute. What is cancer? Available at https://www.cancer.gov/about-cancer/understanding/what-is-cancer.

3. Johns Hopkins Health Review. Understanding inflammation. Spring/Summer

2016. Available at https://www.johnshopkinshealthreview.com/issues/spring-summer-2016/articles/understanding-inflammation.

4. American Institute for Cancer Research. Cancer prevention recommendations. Available at https://www.aicr.org/reduce-your-cancer-risk/recommendations-for-cancer-prevention/.

5. American Cancer Society. Does body weight affect cancer risk? Available at https://www.cancer.org/cancer/cancer-causes/diet-physical-activity/body-weight-and-cancer-risk/effects.html.

6. Hardefeldt PJ, et al. Physical activity and weight loss reduce the risk of breast cancer: a meta-analysis of 139 prospective and retrospective studies. *Clin Breast Cancer.* August 2018; 18(4):e601–12.

7. National Cancer Institute. Artificial sweeteners and cancer. Available at https://www.cancer.gov/about-cancer/causes-prevention/risk/diet/artificial-sweeteners-fact-sheet#is-there-an-association-between-artificial-sweeteners-and-cancer.

8. Norat T, et al. European code against cancer, 4th edition: diet and cancer. *Cancer Epidemiology.* December 2015; 39(1):S56–66.

9. Rajagopala SV, et al. The human microbiome and cancer. *Cancer Prev Res (Phila).* April 10, 2017; 10(4):226–234. Available at https://cancerpreventionresearch.aacrjournals.org/content/10/4/226.long.

10. American Institute for Cancer Research. Get the facts on fiber. Available at https://www.aicr.org/reduce-your-cancer-risk/diet/elements_fiber.html.

11. American Institute for Cancer Research. Alcohol and cancer risk. Available at https://www.aicr.org/reduce-your-cancer-risk/diet/alcohol-and-cancer-risk.html.

12. Alpha-Tocopherol, Beta Carotene Cancer Prevention Study Group. The effect of vitamin E and beta carotene on the incidence of lung cancer and other cancers in male smokers. *N Engl J Med.* April 14, 1994; 330(15):1029–35.

13. American Institute for Cancer Research. Supplements and cancer survivorship. Available at https://www.aicr.org/patients-survivors/healthy-or-harmful/supplements.html.

14. McCullough ML, et al. Circulating vitamin D and colorectal cancer risk: an international pooling project of 17 cohorts. *J Natl Cancer Inst.* February 2019; 111(2):158–69.

15. Mondul AM, et al. Vitamin D and cancer risk and mortality: state of the science, gaps, and challenges. *Epidemiol Rev.* January 2017; 39(1):28–48.

16. American Institute for Cancer Research. Learn more about breast cancer. Available at https://www.aicr.org/learn-more-about-cancer/breast-cancer/.

17. American Institute for Cancer Research. Colorectal cancer continuous update project. Available at https://www.aicr.org/continuous-update-project/colorectal-cancer.html.

18. American Cancer Society. Endometrial cancer risk factors. Available at https://www.cancer.org/cancer/endometrial-cancer/causes-risks-prevention/risk-factors.html.

19. American Institute for Cancer Research. Lifestyle and endometrial cancer risk. Available at https://www.aicr.org/learn-more-about-cancer/endometrial-cancer/index.html.

20. American Institute for Cancer Research. Lifestyle and ovarian cancer risk. Available at https://www.aicr.org/learn-more-about-cancer/ovarian-cancer/index.html.

CHAPTER 7

1. National Institutes of Health. NIH Osteoporosis and Related Bone Diseases National Resource Center. Osteoporosis: peak bone mass in women. Available at https://www.bones.nih.gov/health-info/bone/osteoporosis/bone-mass.

2. Cleveland Clinic. Menopause & osteoporosis. Available at https://my.cleveland clinic.org/health/articles/10091-menopause-osteoporosis.

3. National Osteoporosis Foundation. Osteoporosis fast facts. Available at https://cdn.nof.org/wp-content/uploads/2015/12/Osteoporosis-Fast-Facts.pdf.

4. National Institutes of Health. NIH Osteoporosis and Related Bone Diseases National Resource Center. Oral health and bone disease. Available at https://www.bones.nih.gov/health-info/bone/bone-health/oral-health/oral-health-and-bone-disease.

5. Wright NC, et al. The recent prevalence of osteoporosis and low bone mass in the United States based on bone mineral density at the femoral neck or lumbar spine. *J Bone Miner Res.* 2014; 29(11):2520–26.

6. Abraham A, et al. Premenopausal bone health: osteoporosis in premenopausal women. *Clin Obstet Gynecol.* December 2013; 56(4):722–29.

7. National Institutes of Health. NIH Osteoporosis and Related Bone Diseases National Resource Center. Osteoporosis overview. Available at https://www.bones.nih.gov/health-info/bone/osteoporosis/overview.

8. U.S. Department of Health and Human Services. National Institutes of Health. Office of Dietary Supplements. Calcium. Available at https://ods.od.nih.gov/factsheets/Calcium-HealthProfessional/.

9. Institute of Medicine (US) Standing Committee on the Scientific Evaluation of Dietary Reference Intakes. *Dietary Reference Intakes for Calcium, Phosphorus, Magnesium, Vitamin D, and Fluoride.* Washington, DC: National Academies Press, 1997.

10. U.S. Department of Health and Human Services. National Institutes of Health. Office of Dietary Supplements. Vitamin D. Available at http://ods.od.nih.gov/factsheets/VitaminD-HealthProfessional.

11. Ibid.

12. U.S. Department of Health and Human Services. National Institutes of Health. Office of Dietary Supplements. Dietary supplement fact sheet: magnesium. Available at http://ods.od.nih.gov/factsheets/Magnesium/.

13. Orchard TS, et al. Magnesium intake, bone mineral density, and fractures: results from the Women's Health Initiative observational study. *Am J Clin Nutr.* April 2014; 99(4):926–33.

14. U.S. Department of Health and Human Services. National Institutes of Health. Office of Dietary Supplements. Dietary supplement fact sheet: magnesium. Available at http://ods.od.nih.gov/factsheets/Magnesium/.

15. Institute of Medicine (US) Panel on Micronutrients. *Dietary Reference Intakes for Vitamin A, Vitamin K, Arsenic, Boron, Chromium, Copper, Iodine, Iron, Manganese, Molybdenum, Nickel, Silicon, Vanadium, and Zinc.* Washington, DC: National Academies Press, 2001.

16. Booth SL, et al. Vitamin K intake and bone mineral density in women and men. *Am J Clin Nutr.* February 2003; 77(2): 512–16. Available at https://www.ncbi .nlm.nih.gov/pubmed/12540415.

17. Feskanich D, et al. Vitamin K intake and hip fractures in women: a prospective study. *Am J Clin Nutr.* January 1999; 69(1):74–79.

18. U.S. Department of Health and Human Services. National Institutes of Health. Office of Dietary Supplements. Dietary supplement fact sheet: vitamin K. Available at https://ods.od.nih.gov/factsheets/VitaminK-HealthProfessional/.

19. Malmir H, et al. Vitamin C intake in relation to bone mineral density and risk of hip fracture and osteoporosis: a systematic review and meta-analysis of observational studies. *Br J Nutr.* April 2018; 119(8):847–58.

20. Institute of Medicine (US) Panel on Dietary Antioxidants and Related Compounds. *Dietary Reference Intakes for Vitamin C, Vitamin E, Selenium, and Carotenoids.* Washington, DC: National Academies Press, 2000.

21. U.S. Department of Health and Human Services. National Institutes of Health. Office of Dietary Supplements. Dietary supplement fact sheet: vitamin C. Available at https://ods.od.nih.gov/factsheets/VitaminC-HealthProfessional/.

22. Rizzoli R, et al. Benefits and safety of dietary protein for bone health—an expert consensus paper endorsed by the European Society for Clinical and Economical Aspects of Osteoporosis, Osteoarthritis, and Musculoskeletal Diseases and by the International Osteoporosis Foundation. *Osteoporosis International.* September 2018; 29(9):1933–48.

23. Zheng X, et al. Soy isoflavones and osteoporotic bone loss: a review with an emphasis on modulation of bone remodeling. *J Med Food.* January 1, 2016; 19(1):1–14.

24. Shams-White MM, et al. Animal versus plant protein and adult bone health: a systematic review and meta-analysis from the National Osteoporosis Foundation. *PLoS One.* February 23, 2018; 13(2):e0192459.

25. U.S. Department of Health and Human Services. Physical activity guidelines for Americans, 2nd edition. 2018. Available at https://health.gov/paguidelines /second-edition/.

26. Gaddini GW, et al. Alcohol: a simple nutrient with complex actions on bone in the adult skeleton. *Alcohol Clin Exp Res.* April 2016; 40(4):657–71.

27. Frassetto LA, et al. Adverse effects of sodium chloride on bone in the aging human

population resulting from habitual consumption of typical American diets. *J Nutr.* February 2008; 138(2):419S–22S.

28. Ilich JZ, et al. Higher habitual sodium intake is not detrimental for bones in older women with adequate calcium intake. *Eur J Appl Physiol.* July 2010; 109(4):745–55.

29. National Institutes of Health. NIH Osteoporosis and Related Bone Diseases National Resource Center. Osteoporosis overview. Smoking and bone health. Available at https://www.bones.nih.gov/health-info/bone/osteoporosis/conditions-behaviors/bone-smoking#b.

30. Hallström H. Long-term coffee consumption in relation to fracture risk and bone mineral density in women. *Am J Epidem.* September 15, 2013; 178(6):898–909.

31. U.S. Department of Health and Human Services & U.S. Department of Agriculture. Dietary guidelines for Americans 2015–2020, 8th edition. Caffeine. Available at https://health.gov/dietaryguidelines/2015/guidelines/chapter-2/a-closer-look-at-current-intakes-and-recommended-shifts/#callout-caffeine.

32. Doepker C, Franke K, et al. Key Findings and implications of a recent systematic review of the potential adverse effects of caffeine consumption in healthy adults, pregnant women, adolescents, and children. *Nutrients.* October 2018; 10(10):1536.

33. Centers for Disease Control and Prevention. Does osteoporosis run in your family? Available at https://www.cdc.gov/features/osteoporosis/.

CHAPTER 8

1. Goodman AB, et al. Behaviors and attitudes associated with low drinking water intake among U.S. adults, Food Attitudes and Behaviors Survey, 2007. *Prev Chronic Dis.* April 11, 2013; 10:E51.

2. National Academies of Sciences, Engineering and Medicine. Dietary reference intakes: water, potassium, sodium, chloride, and sulfate. Available at http://www.nationalacademies.org/hmd/Reports/2004/Dietary-Reference-Intakes-Water-Potassium-Sodium-Chloride-and-Sulfate.aspx.

3. Mayo Clinic. Dehydration. Available at https://www.mayoclinic.org/diseases-conditions/dehydration/symptoms-causes/syc-20354086.

4. Emedicinehealth. Dehydration in adults. Available at https://www.emedicinehealth.com/dehydration_in_adults/article_em.htm#what_causes_dehydration_in_adults.

5. Killer SC, et al. No evidence of dehydration with moderate daily coffee intake: a counterbalanced cross-over study in a free-living population. *PLoS One.* January 9, 2014; 9(1):e84154.

6. Academy of Nutrition and Dietetics. Benefits of coffee. Available at https://bit.ly/2VbHGq3.

7. Khan N & Mukhtar H. Tea polyphenols in promotion of human health. *Nutrients.* December 25, 2018; 11(1):39.

8. Hu FB & Malik VS. Sugar-sweetened beverages and risk of obesity and type 2 diabetes: epidemiologic evidence. *Physiol Behav.* April 26, 2010; 100(1):47–54.

9. Centers for Disease Control and Prevention. Get the facts: sugar-sweetened beverages and consumption. Available at https://www.cdc.gov/nutrition/data-statistics /sugar-sweetened-beverages-intake.html.

10. U.S. Department of Health and Human Services. National Institute of Diabetes and Digestive and Kidney Diseases. Non-alcoholic fatty liver disease & NASH. Available at https://www.niddk.nih.gov/health-information/liver-disease /nafld-nash.

11. Asgari-Taee F, et al. Association of sugar sweetened beverages consumption with non-alcoholic fatty liver disease: a systematic review and meta-analysis. *Eur J Nutr.* August 2019; 58(5):1759–69.

12. Ma J, et al. Sugar-sweetened beverage, diet soda, and fatty liver disease in the Framingham Heart Study cohorts. *J Hepatol.* August 2015; 63(2):462–69. Available at https://www.journal-of-hepatology.eu/article/S0168-8278(15)00240-8 /fulltext.

13. O'Keefe EL, et al. Alcohol and CV health: Jekyll and Hyde J-curves. *Prog Cardiovasc Dis.* May–June 2018; 61(1):68–75.

14. U.S. Department of Health and Human Services & U.S. Department of Agriculture. Dietary guidelines for Americans 2015–2020, 8th edition. Appendix 9. Alcohol. Available at https://health.gov/dietaryguidelines/2015/guidelines /appendix-9/.

15. Ashley MJ. Morbidity in alcoholics: evidence for accelerated development of physical disease in women. *Arch Intern Med.* July 1977; 137(7):883–87.

16. Centers for Disease Control and Prevention. Alcohol and public health. Fact sheets—excessive alcohol use and risks to women's health. Available at https:// www.cdc.gov/alcohol/fact-sheets/womens-health.htm.

17. Alcohol.org. Alcohol use demographics and treatment statistics. Available at https://www.alcohol.org/statistics-information/comparing-demographics/.

18. Grant BF, et al. Prevalence of 12-month alcohol use, high-risk drinking, and DSM-IV alcohol use disorder in the United States, 2001–2002 to 2012–2013: results from the National Epidemiologic Survey on Alcohol and Related Conditions. *JAMA Psychiatry.* September 2017; 74(9):911–23.

19. Women's Recovery. Signs of alcoholism in women. Available at https://www .womensrecovery.com/24-signs-alcoholism-women/.

20. National Institutes of Health. National Institute of Alcohol Abuse and Alcoholism. Harmful interactions. Available at https://www.niaaa.nih.gov/publications /brochures-and-fact-sheets/harmful-interactions-mixing-alcohol-with-medicines.

21. Mayo Clinic. Alcohol use disorder. Available at https://www.mayoclinic.org /diseases-conditions/alcohol-use-disorder/symptoms-causes/syc-20369243.

CHAPTER 9

1. Bellettiere J, et al. Sedentary behavior and cardiovascular disease in older women: the OPACH study. *J Am Coll Cardio.* February 19, 2019; 139(8):1036–46.

2. Burd NA, et al. Dietary protein quantity, quality, and exercise are key to healthy living: a muscle-centric perspective across the lifespan. *Front Nutr.* June 6, 2019; 6:83.

3. Agostini D, et al. Muscle and bone health in postmenopausal women: role of protein and vitamin D supplementation combined with exercise training. *Nutrients.* August 16, 2018; 10(8):1103.

4. Burd NA, et al. Dietary protein quantity, quality, and exercise are key to healthy living: a muscle-centric perspective across the lifespan. *Front Nutr.* June 6, 2019; 6:83.

5. Anderson LJ, et al. Sex differences in muscle wasting. *Adv Exp Med Biol.* December 10, 2017; 1043:153–97.

6. Hamrick MW, et al. Fatty infiltration of skeletal muscle: mechanisms and comparisons with bone marrow adiposity. *Front Endocrinol (Lausanne).* June 20, 2016; 7:69.

7. Atherton PJ & Smith K. Muscle protein synthesis in response to nutrition and exercise. *J Physiol.* March 1, 2012; 590(5):1049–57.

8. U.S. Department of Health and Human Services. National Institutes of Health. National Heart, Lung, and Blood Institute. Physical activity and your heart. Available at https://www.nhlbi.nih.gov/health-topics/physical-activity-and-your-heart.

9. Saint-Maurice PF, et al. Association of leisure-time physical activity across the adult life course with all-cause and cause-specific mortality. *JAMA Netw Open.* 2019; 2(3):e190355.

10. Kline CE, et al. Consistently high sports/exercise activity is associated with better sleep quality, continuity, and depth in midlife women: the SWAN sleep study. *Sleep.* September 1, 2013; 36(9):1279–88.

11. Mayo Clinic. Night sweats. Available at https://www.mayoclinic.org/symptoms/night-sweats/basics/definition/sym-20050768.

12. Avis NE, et al. Duration of menopausal vasomotor symptoms over the menopause transition. *JAMA Intern Med.* April 1, 2015; 175(4):531–39.

13. Bailey TG, et al. Exercise training reduces the acute physiological severity of postmenopausal hot flushes. *J Physiol.* December 15, 2015; 594(3):657–67.

14. Berin E, et al. Resistance training for hot flushes in postmenopausal women: a randomised controlled trial. *Maturitas.* August 2019; 126:55–60.

15. Lambiase MJ & Thurston RC. Physical activity and sleep among midlife women with vasomotor symptoms. *Menopause.* September 2013; 20(9):946–52.

16. Biglia N, et al. Non-hormonal strategies for managing menopausal symptoms in cancer survivors: an update. *Ecancermedicalscience.* March 11, 2019; 13:909.

17. Smith RL, et al. Does quitting smoking decrease the risk of midlife hot flashes? A longitudinal analysis. *Maturitas.* September 2015; 82(1):123–27.

18. Stanford KI & Goodyear LJ. Exercise and type 2 diabetes: molecular mechanisms regulating glucose uptake in skeletal muscle. *Adv Physiol Educ.* December 2014; 38(4):308–14.

19. Lee, J et al. Resistance training for glycemic control, muscular strength, and lean body mass in old type 2 diabetic patients: a meta-analysis. *Diabetes Ther.* June 2017; 8(3):459–73.

20. Thomas RJ, et al. Exercise-induced biochemical changes and their potential influence on cancer: a scientific review. *Br J Sports Med.* April 2017; 51(8):640–44.

21. Won J, et al. Semantic memory activation after acute exercise in healthy older adults. *J Intl Neuropsychol Soc.* July 2019; 25(6):557–68.

22. ten Brinke LF, et al. Aerobic exercise increases hippocampal volume in older women with probable mild cognitive impairment: a 6-month randomised controlled trial. *Br J Sports Med.* April 2015; 49(4):248–54.

23. Spartano N, et al. Association of accelerometer-measured light-intensity physical activity with brain volume: the Framingham Heart Study. *JAMA Netw Open.* April 5, 2019; 2(4):e192745. Available at https://jamanetwork.com/journals/jamanetworkopen/fullarticle/2730790.

24. Young SN. How to increase serotonin in the human brain without drugs. *J Psychiatry Neurosci.* November 2007; 32(6):394–99.

25. Choi KW, et al. Assessment of bidirectional relationships between physical activity and depression among adults: a 2-sample Mendelian randomization study. *JAMA Psychiatry.* January 23, 2019; 76(4):399–408.

26. Roman-Blas JA, et al. Osteoarthritis associated with estrogen deficiency. *Arthritis Res Ther.* September 21, 2009; 11(5):241.

27. Allen JM, et al. Exercise alters gut microbiota composition and function in lean and obese humans. *Med Sci Sports Exerc.* April 2018; 50(4):747–57.

28. Church TS, et al. Changes in weight, waist circumference, and compensatory responses with different doses of exercise among sedentary, overweight postmenopausal women. *PLoS One.* February 18, 2009; 4(2):e4515.

29. U.S. Department of Health and Human Services. Physical activity guidelines for Americans, 2nd edition. 2018. Available at https://health.gov/paguidelines/second-edition/.

30. Mcloud JC, et al. Resistance exercise training as a primary countermeasure to age-related chronic disease. *Front Physiol.* June 6, 2019; 10:645. Available at https://www.frontiersin.org/articles/10.3389/fphys.2019.00645/full.

31. U.S. Department of Health and Human Services. Physical activity guidelines for Americans, 2nd edition. 2018. Available at https://health.gov/paguidelines/second-edition/.

32. Janssen I, et al. Correlates of 15-year maintenance of physical activity in middle-aged women. *Int J Behav Med.* 2014; 21(3):511–18.

33. Wall BT, et al. Aging is accompanied by a blunted muscle protein synthetic response to protein ingestion. *PLoS ONE.* November 4, 2015; 10(11): e0140903.

34. Institute of Medicine. *Dietary Reference Intakes for Energy, Carbohydrate, Fiber,*

Fat, Fatty Acids, Cholesterol, Protein, and Amino Acids. Washington, DC: National Academies Press, 2005.

35. Traylor DA, et al. Perspective: protein requirements and optimal intakes in aging: are we ready to recommend more than the recommended daily allowance? *Adv Nutr.* May 15, 2018; 9(3):171–82.

36. Rizzoli R, et al. The role of dietary protein and vitamin D in maintaining musculoskeletal health in postmenopausal women: a consensus statement from the European Society for Clinical and Economic Aspects of Osteoporosis and Osteoarthritis (ESCEO). *Maturitas.* September 2014; 79(1):122–32.

37. Gregorio L, et al. Adequate dietary protein is associated with better physical performance among post-menopausal women 60–90 years. *J Nutr Health Aging.* May 16, 2014; 18(2):155–60.

38. Pennings B, et al. Exercising before protein intake allows for greater use of dietary protein-derived amino acids for de novo muscle protein synthesis in both young and elderly men. *Am J Clin Nutr.* February 2011; 93(2):322–31.

39. Phillips SM. The impact of protein quality on the promotion of resistance exercise-induced changes in muscle mass. *Nutr Metab (Lond).* September 29, 2016; 13(64).

40. McDonald CK, et al. Lean body mass change over 6 years is associated with dietary leucine intake in an older Danish population. *Br J Nutr.* May 2016; 115(9):1556–62.

41. Paddon-Jones D, et al. Protein and healthy aging. *Am J Clin Nutr.* June 2015; 101(6):1339S–45S.

42. Mamerow MM, et al. Dietary protein distribution positively influences 24-h muscle protein synthesis in healthy adults. *J Nutr.* June 2014; 144(6):876–80.

43. Rizzoli R, et al. The role of dietary protein and vitamin D in maintaining musculoskeletal health in postmenopausal women: a consensus statement from the European Society for Clinical and Economic Aspects of Osteoporosis and Osteoarthritis (ESCEO). *Maturitas.* September 2014; 79(1):122–32.

44. Smith GI, Atherton P, Reeds DN, et al. Omega-3 polyunsaturated fatty acids augment the muscle protein anabolic response to hyperinsulinaemia-hyperaminoacidaemia in healthy young and middle-aged men and women. *Clin Sci (Lond).* September 2011; 121(6):267–78.

45. Cintia LN, et al. Fish-oil supplementation enhances the effects of strength training in elderly women. *Am J Clin Nutr.* February 2012; (95)2:428–36.

46. Mayo Clinic. Statin side effects: weigh the benefits and risks. Available at https://www.mayoclinic.org/diseases-conditions/high-blood-cholesterol/in-depth/statin-side-effects/art-20046013.

CHAPTER 10

1. Bailey RL, et al. Why U.S. adults use dietary supplements. *JAMA Intern Med.* March 11, 2013; 173(5):355–61.

2. U.S. Department of Health and Human Services. National Institutes of Health. Office of Dietary Supplements. Calcium. Available at https://ods.od.nih.gov /factsheets/Calcium-HealthProfessional/.

3. U.S. Department of Health and Human Services. National Institutes of Health. Office of Dietary Supplements. Vitamin D. Available at http://ods.od.nih.gov /factsheets/VitaminD-HealthProfessional.

4. U.S. Department of Health and Human Services. National Institutes of Health. Office of Dietary Supplements. Vitamin B_6. Available at https://ods.od.nih.gov /factsheets/VitaminB6-HealthProfessional/.

5. U.S. Department of Health and Human Services. National Institutes of Health. Office of Dietary Supplements. Vitamin B_{12}. Available at https://ods.od.nih.gov /factsheets/VitaminB12-HealthProfessional/#en24.

6. Institute of Medicine. Dietary Reference Intakes for Vitamin A, Vitamin K, Arsenic, Boron, Chromium, Copper, Iodine, Iron, Manganese, Molybdenum, Nickel, Silicon, Vanadium, and Zinc. Washington, DC: National Academics Press, 2001.

7. U.S. Food and Drug Administration. What you need to know about dietary supplements. Available at https://www.fda.gov/food/buy-store-serve-safe-food/what -you-need-know-about-dietary-supplements.

8. U.S. Department of Health and Human Services & U.S. Department of Agriculture. Dietary guidelines for Americans, 2015–2020, 8th edition. December 2015. Available at https://health.gov/dietaryguidelines/2015/guidelines/.

9. U.S. Department of Health and Human Services & U.S. Department of Agriculture. Scientific report of the 2015 Dietary Guidelines Advisory Committee. Available at https://health.gov/dietaryguidelines/2015-scientific-report/PDFs /Scientific-Report-of-the-2015-Dietary-Guidelines-Advisory-Committee.pdf.

10. U.S. Department of Agriculture, Agricultural Research Service. Nutrient intakes from food and beverages: mean amounts consumed per individual, by gender and age, in the United States, 2013–2014. *What We Eat in America, NHANES.* Available at https://www.ars.usda.gov/ARSUserFiles/80400530/pdf/1314/Table _1_NIN_GEN_13.pdf.

11. U.S. Department of Health and Human Services & U.S. Department of Agriculture. Scientific report of the 2015 Dietary Guidelines Advisory Committee. Available at https://health.gov/dietaryguidelines/2015-scientific-report/PDFs /Scientific-Report-of-the-2015-Dietary-Guidelines-Advisory-Committee.pdf.

12. Kantor ED, et al. Trends in dietary supplement use among U.S. adults from 1999–2012. *JAMA.* October 11, 2016; 316(14):1464–74.

13. U.S. Department of Health and Human Services. National Institutes of Health. Office of Dietary Supplements. Omega-3 fatty acids. Available at https://ods.od .nih.gov/factsheets/Omega3FattyAcids-Consumer/.

14. Ibid.

15. U.S. Department of Agriculture, Agricultural Research Service. Nutrient intakes from food and beverages: mean amounts consumed per individual, by gender and age, in the United States, 2013–2014. *What We Eat in America,*

NHANES. Available at https://www.gars.usda.gov/northeast-area/beltsville-md-bhnrc/beltsville-human-nutrition-research-center/food-surveys-research-group/docs/wweia-data-tables/.

16. World Health Organization & Food and Agriculture Organization. WHO Joint FAO/WHO Expert Consultation on Fats and Fatty Acids in Human Nutrition. WHO; Geneva, Switzerland: 2008. Available at http://www.who.int/nutrition/topics/FFA_interim_recommendations/en/.

17. Miller M, et al. Triglycerides and cardiovascular disease: a scientific statement from the American Heart Association. *Circulation.* May 24, 2011; 123(20):2292–333.

18. U.S. Department of Agriculture, Agricultural Research Service. Nutrient intakes from food and beverages: mean amounts consumed per individual, by gender and age, in the United States, 2013–2014. *What We Eat in America, NHANES.* Available at https://www.gars.usda.gov/northeast-area/beltsville-md-bhnrc/beltsville-human-nutrition-research-center/food-surveys-research-group/docs/wweia-data-tables/.

19. Fischer LM, et al. Dietary choline requirements of women: effects of estrogen and genetic variation. *Am J Clin Nutr.* September 22, 2010; 92(5):1113–19.

20. Gibson GR, et al. Expert consensus document: the International Scientific Association for Probiotics and Prebiotics (ISAPP) consensus statement on the definition and scope of prebiotics. *Nat Rev Gastroenterol Hepatol.* August 2017; 14(8): 491–502.

21. National Institutes of Health. National Library of Medicine. Lactobacillus. Available at https://medlineplus.gov/druginfo/natural/790.html.

22. National Institutes of Health. National Center for Complementary and Integrative Medicine. Probiotics: what you need to know. Available at https://nccih.nih.gov/health/probiotics/introduction.htm.

23. Khalesi S, et al. Effect of probiotics on blood pressure: a systematic review and meta-analysis of randomized, controlled trials. *Hypertension.* July 2014; 64(4):897–903.

24. Skokovic-Sunjic D. Clinical guide to probiotic products available in USA: indications, dosage forms, and clinical evidence to date, 2019 edition. Available at www.usprobioticguide.com.

25. U.S. Food and Drug Administration. Drug safety communication. Available at https://www.fda.gov/drugs/drug-safety-and-availability/fda-drug-safety-communication-low-magnesium-levels-can-be-associated-long-term-use-proton-pump.

26. Freedberg DE, et al. The risks and benefits of long-term use of proton pump inhibitors: expert review and best practice advice from the American Gastroenterology Association. *Gastroenterology.* March 2017; 152(4):706–15.

27. Aroda VR, et al. Long-term metformin use and vitamin B_{12} deficiency in the Diabetes Prevention Program Outcomes Study. *J Clin Endocrinol Metab.* April 2016; 101(4):1754–61.

28. U.S Food and Drug Administration. Mixing medications and dietary

supplement can endanger your health. Available at https://www.fda.gov/consumers/consumer-updates/mixing-medications-and-dietary-supplements-can-endanger-your-health.

CHAPTER 11

1. Reidlinger DP, et al. Resting metabolic rate and anthropometry in older people: a comparison of measured and calculated values. *J Hum Nutr Diet.* February 2015; 28(1):72–78.
2. U.S. Department of Health and Human Services & U.S. Department of Agriculture. 2015–2020 dietary guidelines for Americans. 8th edition. Appendix 2. Estimated calorie needs per day, by age, sex, and physical activity level. Available at https://health.gov/dietaryguidelines/2015/guidelines/appendix-2/.
3. Tucker JM, et al. Physical activity in U.S. adults: compliance with the Physical Activity Guidelines for Americans. *Am J Prev Med.* April 2011; 40(4):454–61.
4. Longo V & Panda S. Fasting, circadian rhythms, and time restricted feeding in healthy lifespan. *Cell Metab.* June 14, 2016; 23(6):1048–59.
5. Gabel K. et al. Effects of 8-hour time restricted feeding on body weight and metabolic disease risk factors in obese adults: a pilot study. *Nutrition and Healthy Aging.* June 15, 2018; 4(4):345–53.
6. Gill S & Panda S. A smartphone app reveals erratic diurnal eating patterns in humans that can be modulated for health benefits. *Cell Metab.* November 3, 2015; 22(5):789–98.
7. Marinac CR, et al. Prolonged nightly fasting and breast cancer risk: findings from NHANES (2009–2010). *Cancer Epidemiol Biomarkers Prev.* April 20, 2015; 24(5):783–89.
8. Marinac CR, et al. Prolonged nightly fasting and breast cancer prognosis. *JAMA Oncol.* August 1, 2016; 2(8):1049–55.
9. Longo V & Panda S. Fasting, circadian rhythms, and time restricted feeding in healthy lifespan. *Cell Metab.* June 14, 2016; 23(6):1048–59.
10. Oldways. Traditional Diets. Available at https://oldwayspt.org/traditional-diets.
11. Salley J, et al. Comparison between human and bite-based methods of estimating caloric intake. *J Acad Nutr Diet.* October 2016; 116(10):1568–77.
12. Gaesser GA. Perspective: refined grains and health: genuine risk, or guilt by association? *Adv Nutr.* May 1, 2019; 10(3):361–71.
13. U.S. Department of Health and Human Services & U.S. Department of Agriculture. Dietary guidelines for Americans. 2015–2020. 8th edition. Available at http://health.gov/dietaryguidelines/2015/guidelines/.
14. Interview with Dr. Woods. June 2009.
15. Urban LE, et al. Energy contents of frequently ordered restaurant meals and comparison with human energy requirements and U.S. Department of Agri-

culture Database Information: a multisite randomized study. *J Acad Nutr Diet.* April 2016; 116(4):590–98.

CHAPTER 12

1. Mejia SB, et al. A meta-analysis of 46 studies identified by the FDA demonstrates that soy protein decreases circulating LDL and total cholesterol concentrations in adults. *J Nutr.* June 2019; 149(6):968–81.
2. Arab L, et al. Lower depression scores among walnut consumers in NHANES. *Nutrients.* January 26, 2019; 11(2):275.
3. Holscher H, et al. Walnut consumption alters the gastrointestinal microbiota, microbially derived secondary bile acids, and health markers in healthy adults: a randomized controlled trial. *J Nutrition.* June 2018; 148(6):861–67.
4. Xiao Y, et al. Effect of nut consumption on vascular endothelial function: a systematic review and meta-analysis of randomized controlled trials. *Clin Nutr.* April 20, 2017; 37(8):831–39.
5. Buendia B, et al. Regular yogurt intake and risk of cardiovascular disease among hypertensive adults. *Am J Hypertension.* May 2018; 31(5):557–65.

INDEX

ABOUT THE AUTHORS

HILLARY WRIGHT, MED, RDN, is a registered dietitian and the author of *The PCOS Diet Plan* and *The Prediabetes Diet Plan*. She is the director of nutrition counseling for the Domar Center for Mind/Body Health at Boston IVF, a Harvard-affiliated fertility treatment center. She also works part-time as a senior nutritionist at the Dana-Farber Cancer Institute in Boston, Massachusetts, and is a founding member of the nutrition technology company Good Measures LLC.

ELIZABETH WARD, MS, RDN, is a registered dietitian with more than thirty years of experience counseling patients and writing about nutrition and health. She is an experienced recipe developer and food photographer and the author or coauthor of several books, including *Super Nutrition After 50, Live Longer and Better*, and *Expect the Best: Your Guide to Healthy Eating Before, During, and After Pregnancy*. Ward blogs about a healthy lifestyle at betteristhenewperfect.com.

Available from

HILLARY WRIGHT

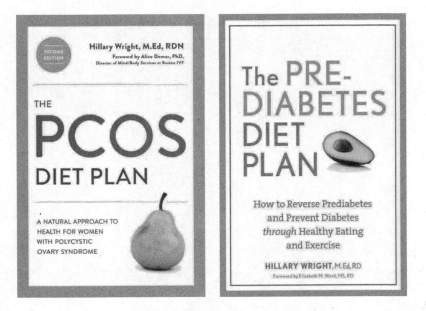

Available wherever books are sold